HEALED FROM
SCHIZOPHRENIA

HEALED FROM SCHIZOPHRENIA

A BIOGRAPHY OF THE EPIC ACCOUNT OF JILL'S JOURNEY

DELINE TAN

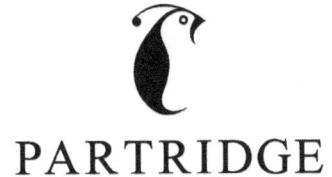

PARTRIDGE

To order additional copies of this book, contact
Toll Free +65 3165 7531 (Singapore)
Toll Free +60 3 3099 4412 (Malaysia)
orders.singapore@partridgepublishing.com

www.partridgepublishing.com/singapore

CONTENTS

ENDORSEMENTS

In *Healed from Schizophrenia,* the author, Deline Tan, gives a heartwarming account of Jill's childhood experiences till adulthood. Through the clear narrative account, the reader is inspired to God's precious anointing of healing, and the special touches on Jill's life.

The book is for all who long to hear God's voice, and to come into a saving knowledge and acceptance of the Savior of the world, Jesus Christ.

This is my prayer that we will recognize any harm that will come into our lives, to find release in the Scriptures, and receive God's blessings, through the Christian men and women, who are available for counsel and prayer.

Dr. Suraja Raman
Missionary/Teaching faculty in theological schools in Asia & Africa
Researcher

Healed from Schizophrenia helps one to understand the debilitating effects of a mental illness such as schizophrenia, and how it affects every facet of life from the emotional to the social life of the individual, and yes, including one's own walk with Jesus. Yet, more importantly, the account on the journal entries reveal a more important truth, which is the Providence of God. How God will take the life of a broken vessel and fashion it into something beautiful that would only result in His glory. Yes, it is truly the faithfulness of a loving God revealed as you read through the pages, and especially the journal entries of the past decades.

David Chan Soon Onn
Social Worker

Reading *"Healed from Schizophrenia"* peels open the protagonist childhood years, adolescence and adulthood, as it expresses who she was and what she has been through. Her story of resilience and recovery throughout the difficult years of physical and mental pain uncovers the painful times of helplessness and hopelessness. Then again, her firm believe in God and to know that without God she is nothing, she courageously braved the paths of hurts, bitterness, anguish and despair. Through the grace of God, she is where she is today.

Frank M.
Programme Manager
Caregivers Alliance Ltd

This book is a sincere attempt to recall Jill's life, painful as it still is, suffering numerous relapses of schizophrenia from young adult to her fifties, but never, never giving up on searching for an answer and a breakthrough from God. It will bring hope to many with or without mental health issues, to know that we are never alone in our struggles, that we can learn to live purposefully and go beyond a merely existential mindset, even with a severe mental deficit that hogs us in our lives. By writing this biography, Deline is giving glory to Christ Jesus, who saves a life of despair to a life of hope. I count it a privilege to endorse this courageous attempt by the author to connect the dots in Jill's life. This book also challenges us to write our own story prayerfully, so as to find meaning out of the chaos of our past and give ourselves a second chance to live anew for the rest of our lives. This is such an important perspective in our current struggle with the Covid pandemic, which makes our tomorrow a greater uncertainty.

Florence Ng
Co-founder of Turning Point Halfway House
(A recovery program for women drug addicts)

FOREWORD

I am always eager to read about the transformation which God does in someone's life. When Deline Tan approached me about writing a foreword for her biography, I was interested to see what God had done in her life over the years. Deline had attended some of the Bible School classes I have taught over the years and I wanted to know how God had worked in and through her.

In her biography, Deline takes the reader through the early years of Jill's obstacles and trials. Through many setbacks along the way, Jill is forced to lean on God and His power. In the end, it is refreshing to see that despite all the problems which faced her, she was able to come out victorious by God's power.

Deline Tan's book delves into the discouragement that can come from waiting in years for an answer. She vulnerably shares about Jill's difficulties over the years. She explores the ups and downs of Christian life, but then in the end she admits that through everything

God has always been faithful. It was encouraging to see the lessons which she learned in the midst of her struggles. It was encouraging to see that God can use even those things which the world would consider to be negative events in our life to bring about His glory and His healing.

Rev Dr. Margaret B. Seaward
Lecturer at Asia Theological Center / Pastor

PREFACE

Life is a struggle if we have gone through the ups and downs of life. It is even more discouraging if all dams broke lose when we don't know how to recover from the trauma that we faced. It is even more dampened if all around us, we do not get the support that we need from our peers or family members. How are we faring if all around us are chaos and despair? How do we face our tomorrows if we are discouraged with what is happening around us? Does life seem fair when we try our utmost best to get what we wanted but failed miserably? How do we progress forward when all our baggage seems so heavy? Do we find hope at the end of the tunnel? Do we feel loved in spite of all our setbacks? How do we move forward when all around us seems so hopeless?

One thing is true in life when we look beyond ourselves and try to see the rainbow at the end of our road block. Do we see colours, or a mash of faded colours and everything is so unclear? Whatever you are facing, know that life is beautiful and at the end of it all, God will always break through for us if we look to God and get our solutions from Him. God is who He is and He can mend broken lives. Have you found your answers in all your struggles? God is looking for you if you will only allow Him to get hold of your life. God is who He is and you just have to reach out to Him and He will take care of all your pains and struggles. Only look to Him and all will be well and at ease.

Deline Tan
Author

PART 1

CHILDHOOD & ADOLESCENT YEARS

Jill Quah, a delicate four-year-old, was crying incessantly on a daily basis. What was her problem? Well, her mother, Madame Soh, seemed to punish her for every little action she did. Jill would climb the chairs and tables and turned everything upside down within her reach. She was full of activity. She was a vibrant kid. Playing outside her house, she would dig sand and mud and drench herself all over. Returning home with her dirty clothes covered in mud, Madame Soh would cane Jill for her dirty attire and sent her crying all day. If she wasn't beaten for 'naughty' play, then it would be for eating too much.

"How do you think you can take your dinner with all the junk that you are eating right now?" Madame Soh chided.

"I'm hungry now, but I will eat again later at dinner," Jill replied.

"You spoilt little brad, you ought to receive caning."

Madame Soh reached for the cane. Little Jill would run around the house with big mama running all over the house with her.

"You naughty little kid, you can't have dinner if you were to eat now." Madame Soh yelled.

"I'm sorry Mummy, but I am hungry."

Such a scene was a normal occurrence for Jill. Or Jill would put on her innocent look and chat continuously with her paternal grandmother. Grandma Ku would offer Jill some sweets. Jill secretly kept the sweets to herself, fearing her mother's discovery.

"The weather is so cold today, Grandma. It rained all day,"

Grandma Ku would tell Jill stories about herself when young, and Jill would tell her about her outdoor adventure—how she would pick the colourful flowers and fall into the muddy water accidentally.

Jill was active in sports. When she turned 10, she was involved in the school sport team and came in as champion in the one hundred metre race. High jump and long jump were next to her favourite sports, and she came in second in high jump when she was 12. Her active demeanour saw her winning trophies for over three years, from when she was 10 to 12 years old.

She was very talkative and vibrant, but in class she would fight with her classmates. "This is mine," Jill would yell at her classmates and fight over her pencil.

"This is not yours, but mine..." Her classmates would yell back in return.

Fighting was a usual occurrence in class. Jill became overtly active in class to the extent that she failed to pay attention to her lessons. She failed miserably in her grades and would get red marks for all subjects. She would cringe in fear each time she had to hand her report card to her dad. However, her dad was lenient towards her and didn't utter a single word to reprimand her. But although Dad never scolded Jill, he never spent time with Jill in her growing-up years, as he was busy at work as a shop assistant. She never knew her dad all her life, as he showed no interest in her growing-up years.

Standing outside her class for mischievous behaviour, Jill would be humiliated by her teacher as a normal punishment. When she disobeyed, her teacher made her suck a pacifier in class.

"Can't you understand how to do this simple maths?" Her teacher yelled at Jill.

"Quit school if you have to, as you are so stupid," The teacher echoed.

Jill was abused by her teacher daily, as she was deemed to be of no earthly good. Her delicate and tender childhood was slain by her poor performance in school. She never became a confident person, but was humiliated with childhood wounds and hurts. She grew up hurting and suffered an inferiority complex.

The pain from her childhood began to crystalize in her inner emotions when she became an adult. Her inferior adulthood was the result of her inner fear as a child. The inner struggles were the pain of unspoken needs. She could not have what she wanted, and life seemed to be so unfair. It traumatised her as an unheard child. Where were the talents that God gave her to fulfil her dreams? Where were the young girl's unspoken needs? She would embrace love, but she never knew what it was like to be loved. There were many promises in her, but how could she attain the kind of life with the gifted talents that God had given her?

Why would all the talents be buried inside? Wouldn't it manifest itself to show God's splendour? Couldn't she hear an innocent voice speak? Where were all the rewards, if any, if she didn't know how to attain them? Let the child in her speak. Let the creation hold back and allow the wrath of God to destroy those who destroyed the child in Jill. Let God arise and the enemy be shattered. May God see her potential, as she accepts what the future holds in spite of a broken childhood. God can heal the soul and in His perfect timing, He will make good what she had lost as a child.

At 15, Jill told God she wanted to be happy and never have to grow up. She could not imagine herself dressing up in office attire and going to work. She wanted to wear knee-length socks, wear mini-skirts, and be an exercise instructor. She loved sports, as she was sporty, active, and vibrant.

One day, Jill was in her room together with her second sister, Jane.

"How would you like to experience the top of the world, Jill?" Jane asked.

"At the top of the world? How?" Jill replied.

"Here, look. Step onto this stool, and you can climb to the top of the wardrobe. From there you can experience the top of the world feeling."

Jill was thrilled with what her sister told her, and she climbed onto the top of the wardrobe. While up there, Jane removed the stool and left Jill hanging in the balance. She couldn't climb down, and to Jill's horror, she jumped down from the eight-foot wardrobe but was not hurt.

"Phew …! You managed to jump down? How brave of you," Jane said.

This was the beginning of Jill's journey. Jane would humiliate her, attack her, and make her life miserable.

"You can't take the egg!" Jane shouted as Jill was having her breakfast.

"You are so greedy. Just drink your milo and stop eating the bread too." Jane outrageously attacked Jill.

"Why can't I have the egg and the bread?' Jill asked.

"Because you are a glutton, and I don't like seeing you eating," Jane yelled.

In the fit of Jane's anger, she snatched back the egg and bread and left Jill crying.

Jill would cry incessantly, and kept her emotions to herself. She didn't tell her mother the injustice shown to her by her sister. Day in and day out, Jane would bully Jill. Jill would feel miserable and down-hearted, and her countenance fell. Jill began to suffer from low self-esteem, and an inferiority complex. She did not know how to vent her fear. And she was always feeling sorry for herself.

Jane, too, would quarrel with her mother, and she talked to no one as she developed a hatred for all her family members. She quit school at secondary three level and did not complete her education. She was constantly harassing Jill and caused a deep scar in Jill's life.

Jill turned to no one for help and did not tell her parents about the situation. She was introverted and helpless. She did not know how to help herself and was fearful. She would later in her life develop a sickness like schizophrenia. All her rationalised reasons for living would vanish away. She lost her sense of reality and would not be able to rationalise things.

Life was full of trauma for Jill, as she faced two incidences that marred her entire life. One was when she jumped down from the wardrobe, and the other was during her army days when fear triggered an attack in her life. Jill joined the army when she was 18. While she was new in the army camp, the staff brought fear to her when they painted a horrendous situation of the camp. They said the army drivers were horrid people, and they told her that they would bring harm and disaster to her. She was horrified and was really fearful about the whole matter. However, this incident brought fear and anxiety in her later life— she was really fearful and anxious when things didn't go her way.

"Why is my computer going wrong?" Jill would panic when something went wrong. "Why is it that everyone is going against me?" She would be anxious and really fearful. She feared being late for appointments and would be frantic that people would wait for her. Anxiety and anxiousness would grip her, and she would be very fearful.

Her sad fate didn't just happen to her on account of her second sister, but her brother, Dave, too, would attack her.

"Get out of my way, you jerk," Dave would humiliate Jill. "Let me not see you again trying to eat these fruits," he would threaten. "Don't show your face again. I don't want to see you," Dave would slanderously attack Jill. "You are so useless. Never come to any good."

Jill would silently suffer such remarks and she was speechless. She was defenceless and alone. She would cry in the night and sorrow would drench her soul deeply.

Apart from her siblings treating her badly, she, too, faced her mother, who would be very unkind to her. "Stop eating the fish; there are others before you," she would say to Jill. "Wash the plates." Such were the remarks that her mum would constantly nag at Jill.

"Jill, you can't do this, you can't do that!" Her mum would echo to her. In her siblings' squabbles, her mum would take sides in favour of the other siblings rather than be merciful to Jill. She was always the odd one out. She was the black sheep in the family. The constant conflicts she faced drew her away from her family. She was distance and cold. She talked to no one in the family. She faced life all on her own. Jill drew away from everyone and kept to herself, and she began to suffer from depression.

Jill began to live a world of her own, where the whole world was her enemy. She hardly had any friends as she isolated herself. She was hostile, rude, and arrogant. She kept to herself, with no friends, and no relationship with her family. She quarreled with her elder brother Dave who provoked and attacked her. She could not bear the humiliation and fought back. It was a night mare as she would constantly engage in fights.

One day, in the heat of the sunny day, Jill found herself in a difficult situation, where God asked her to apologise to Dave. She did, and her relationship with him took a turn. He no longer bullied her and they could relate again. At the lowest point of her life, God delivered her, healed Jill of her emotion, changed and transformed her. As her world fell apart when she did not know how to handle the situations, God broke through.

Life goes on as usual for Jill, but she was traumatised with fear. The sun would not set without Jill suffering the pain of abandonment.

"Will you get out of the bathroom as I need to bathe now?" Her third sister Jolene would yell.

"This is not fair; I came in first." Jill would protest.

"I'm late for my appointment, and besides you have plenty of time later to bathe." Jolene added.

Jill fought with Jolene since young, even until the adulthood. It was always a petty issue that saw the mountain in a mole hill. "Can you be more considerate. I want to sleep now. Please off the light." Jill asked.

"It is still early; besides I'm not done with my reading." Jolene replied.

"I said off the light now." Jill yelled.

"Why should I do what you said? Who do you think you are?"

By this time Jill switched off the light, and Jolene shouted, "On the light now!"

Jolene challenged her, while Jill went to her bed, but Jolene continued to yell, and went to switch on the light.

By this time Jill was agitated, got up from her bed and tried to hit Jolene but missed her. Jolene defended herself, went out of the room and told her mum about Jill and the quarrel.

Mum came to the room and shouted, "Why are you so disrespectful towards your sister. She wants to read, why should you off the light? Now, get out of your bed."

"I want to sleep. Can you ask her to stop reading?" Jill protested.

Mum switched on the light and warned Jill, "Don't you dare off the light again."

Jill buried her head into the pillow, but she was furious.

"Don't you dare to behave in this manner again." Mum chided.

There were many fights between Jill and Jolene, and their mother always spoke for Jolene, and put Jill down. She would not see Jill's reasoning, but she sided Jolene no matter what the fight was all about. Jill felt the injustice to her and was always the victim of her mother's blame.

Jill grew up in the middle-class family and was a very energetic and playful child. She talked a lot and her speech was quick and fast. There was no pause in her speech. She rattled through every word and every sentence. She played all day and would not study. She would walk about bare footed and play outside the house. She came from a big family, as she has six siblings, and her family stayed together with her uncle's (Jill father's brother) family in a huge bungalow purchased by her grandfather. Her uncle had five children and they all ate and played in the same house. She grew up together with her cousins in both their sad and happy times. Her cousins would play with her and the youngest cousin would relate freely with her and teach her things, as well as share the gospel with her when she was about 12 years old. She became a Christian and attended Katong Presbyterian Church. She would attend Sunday School and joined the Presbyterian Youth Fellowship. She was close to her cousins and they had a great time playing together. They would eat together at a big table for lunch and dinner, and her mum or aunty would cook a big pot of rice for 12 children. Chinese New Year was always very special for Jill, as they would celebrate when her mum and aunty would cook many good dishes to offer to the deity on the eve of Chinese New Year. Then the children would receive Ang Pows (red packets) from her father and uncle, and they would gamble away. They wore new clothes and really had much fun and would go for movies and ate satay. The New Year's eve saw fire crackers exploded after worship to the deity. The whole atmosphere of Chinese New Year was very lively and bubbly, as Jill really enjoyed herself together with her family and cousins.

In their free time, Jill and her cousins would play chess and other games, and table-tennis was their usual game as they had a table-tennis table. Jill played often in the table-tennis as well as badminton. They would play hide and seek and they grew together in harmonious setting and Jill really enjoyed her years playing and growing up with her cousins.

Jill accepted Christ when she was 12 years old, after her cousin shared with her the gospel. On one blissful evening, Jill walked into Katong Presbyterian Church where they hosted a Coffee House. There was loud music and hotdogs and burgers were served.

Jill was introduced to a counsellor named Wendy. "How do you do? Nice meeting you." Wendy said.

"I'm fine, thank you. Nice meeting you too." Jill replied.

"Is this your first time in a church?" Wendy asked.

"Yes, that's right. This is my first time."

"That's great. Nice to have you here."

"Thanks!" Jill added.

"Do you like something to eat? A burger perhaps?" Wendy asked.

"OK sure. I wouldn't mind one."

"How about drinks?"

"Yes, a coke will do. Thanks!"

After Jill had eased herself in a comfortable place with a coke and burger, she felt a sense of peace that enveloped her.

"How do you like the music?" Wendy asked.

"It's great. This is the first time that I listen to a Christian music." Jill added.

"Wow … this is so wonderful. How do you like it?"

"It's amazing."

"What standard at school are you in right now? Wendy asked.

"Primary Six."

"Ok, so you're 12 years old?"

"Yes, I will be when I hit my next birthday in July."

"Wonderful. Now may I ask if you have ever heard about the person named Jesus?"

"Yes, my cousin shared with me about Jesus before."

"Oh, this is so wonderful. Jesus is a Son of God and if you accept Jesus you shall be saved." Wendy added.

"Whoa … tell me more."

"Two thousand years ago, Jesus came to this world to identify Himself with mankind. He came to this world to redeem us to God as we are all sinners. He came with the purpose of saving you and me. He died a horrible death on the cross, but three days later He rose from the dead."

"This is so incredible."

"God loves us so much that He sent Jesus to come to this world to set us free from our sins. Do you believe that you are a sinner?"

"Yeah … I think so!"

"Sin separate us from God. But God sent Jesus to pay for the penalty of our sins. When you believe in Him, you shall be saved."

Jill was silent.

"Jesus came to this world to identify Himself with men. We are all sinners and deserve to go to hell, but Jesus loves us so much that He was willing to pay the penalty for our sins. He came to this earth for you and me, to die on the cross to save mankind."

Jill was still silent.

"I like to introduce this person Jesus to you. If you believe you are a sinner, Jesus has already paid for your penalty by dying on the cross. Do you believe in Him?"

Wendy continued, "Jesus is reaching out to you now, and if you believe in Him for what He has done for you, you shall be saved."

Jill was attentive and thought deeply.

Wendy asked again, "Do you want to receive Jesus into your heart right now?"

"I ... I ...!

"Don't worry. Jesus is with you now. He invites you into His heart. As you believe in Him, you shall be saved."

Wendy nudged at Jill, "Do you want to accept Jesus into your life right now?"

"Yes! If Jesus died for my sin, I want to believe in Him."

"Great! Do you really want to accept Jesus into your life?"

"Yes! I want this Jesus."

"Ok, good. Then repeat this prayer after me. Dear Lord Jesus, I thank you that you died for my sins on the cross and now as I believe in You, I shall be saved. Thank you for forgiving me for all my sins, as I now receive You into my heart. In Jesus most precious name I pray. Amen!" "Congratulations, you are now a child of God, Jill"

"Thank you Wendy for your prayers. I am glad that I now believe in Jesus."

"This is so wonderful. I will help you to study the Bible, as it is the Word of God. Can I visit you one of these days?"

"Urr … urr … ok!"

"Great! I will call you and let you know when I can visit you."

"Ok thanks!" Jill was delighted.

The glow on Jill's face was visible that she has finally met God and accepted Jesus. She went away from the meeting completely blessed.

As promised, Wendy visited Jill to do Bible Study. She went to her house where she was gladly accepted. Wendy asked, "Can I pray for you first."

"Yes, you may."

"Dear Lord Jesus, I commit Jill into your loving hand, that as she studies the Word, she shall be blessed and understand it without any difficulty. In Jesus name I pray. Amen!" Okay, you can find the New Testament in the second half of the Bible. We shall study the Book of John for a start. You can share the Bible with me. Ok, let's read The Gospel of John, Chapter One, verse one.

'In the beginning was the Word, and the Word was with God, and the Word was God.' (NKJV)

Slowly they began to read verse by verse, until verses 19 to 22, where Wendy expounded the truth to Jill. 'Verse 19 – Now this is the testimony of John, when the Jews sent priests and Levites from Jerusalem to ask him, "Who are You?"' 'Verse 20 – He confessed and did not deny but confessed, "I am not the Christ". Verse 21 – And they asked him, "What then? Are you Elijah?" He said, "I am not" "Are you the Prophet?" And he answered, "No." Verse 22 – Then they said to him, "Who are you, that we may give an answer to those who sent us? What do you say about yourself?"'(NKJV)

As Wendy went through the verses with Jill, the Word was crystal clear and affirmative. Jill thoroughly understood who the people said John was and his role as John the Baptist. After the Bible Study, it was time to pray, and Wendy urged Jill to pray. However, Jill just stood there silent, unwilling to pray. Wendy urged her again to pray; but Jill stood still without a word. This pattern that Jill displayed for not praying went on for a few sessions of the Bible Study, until Wendy finally gave up doing Bible Study with Jill. However, Jill did not slip back on the church, as she attended Katong Presbyterian Church. Jill would see Wendy once in a while in the church, but the mentorship discontinued. During this time Jill was very unsteady in attending the church, as she would skip church at times and some other times, she would attend church.

However, Jill joined the Presbyterian Youth Fellowship (PYF) and grew in her Christian walk there. The music was soothing, chairs were arranged in a circle, a group of about 15 youths would come together to sing songs, play games, share their testimonies, have the Word of God shared by the leader, and praying for one another.

Worshipping the Lord at PYF was the norm that the youths met. Once a week on a week night, they would gather and have fun together. Sometimes they play musical chairs, where an item would be passed around, and when the music stopped, the one who held the item would have to do a forfeit. When it came to Jill's forfeit, she would bravely put a front, and tried her best to mimic the sound of a dog or cat; or at other times, she would be caught to do some singing or acting.

Rage & Anger

When Jill was 15, she developed an inexplicable and uncontrollable reaction towards people. She shouted and yelled at anybody who stepped on her toes. Her outbursts were really bad until in her adult years, God removed it from her. She did not know how to build relationship with her family members, as well as people in the society, as she does not have best-friends in school. In fact, during her schooling years, she was under attack and bullied by her schoolmates. Her teachers, too, hated and mobbed Jill by asking me to leave school, as she was slow in learning. One of the teachers hit and slapped her when she did not know how to do her mathematics.

Jill was very active and talkative while in her primary school years, as she would disrupt others and was very inattentive in class. The reason why she did not do well in school was because she was playful and could not be still in class. She was always talking and was never focused on her studies. She developed an inferiority complex and fear for men because of the negative upbringing in her life. Her negative childhood brought about her inability to relate appropriately with others, as she was always talking without listening.

PART 2

ADULTHOOD

Jill's School Life

Life in school was a routine, as nothing spectacular happened. Jill failed in all her exams, as she did not know how to study. She had few friends in class and never had a best friend. She did not participate in sports because no one knew her talent as she was transferred to Chai Chee Secondary School. As she joined the sports team, she did not win any prize because she did not train. She failed her GCE 'O' Level and repeated at a different private school at Saint Francis School. She had a good time with her classmates, as they would often party at one of the classmates' houses. She had fond memories there as she enjoyed her classmates and was quite close to them. Today, she is still in touch with one of her classmates. They would often go for meals and fellowship together.

Jill's best time and favorite subject in school was PE (Physical Education). She loved sports and was active. Next to PE was Literature and English, her next favorite subjects. She was poor in Mathematics, but loved Biology. She did not excel well in school as she was a very poor student. She felt deceived that her school subjects did not help her in her future work life, therefore she hated to study and was looking forward to work in society.

Church Attendance

Jill left Katong Presbyterian Church in 1986, after two years of recovery from mental illness. A friend brought her to Chen Li Presbyterian Church and she remained there because of the adult fellowship that she joined and enjoyed. She would have regular bible study in the fellowship, as they met every Sunday. They had fun time together, as they sang, shared messages, played games, and were accountable to one another. They would go for carols and visit households during Christmas eve yearly.

Jill left Chen Li Presbyterian Church after she found herself wandering at the adult fellowship. She went to Bedok Methodist Church in 2000 as a friend invited her to join him in the church. It was a very trying time for Jill there, as she had no relationship with anyone and she was all by herself. God later asked her to attend Faith Community Baptist Church (FCBC).

She was there from 1992 to 2000. She grew spiritually there and attended cell groups. It was during this time that God helped to prune and transform Jill into His likeness, as she nursed a still troubled mind because of schizophrenia. In the cell group, she could not relate with the members and found herself introverted and very much keeping to herself. She could not relate and suffered inner loneliness. It was not until the last cell group she attended that she was delivered from loneliness. She could relate to the people there, and it seemed that she had found her cell group, but God interrupted and asked her to join Tabernacle of Holiness. She left in 2000 from FCBC and joined Tabernacle of Holiness.

It was there at Tabernacle of Holiness that the Lord trained her how to handle relationship and to build rapport with people. She could not relate with the Senior Pastor, as he was not approachable, and there was a barrier between them. She did not know how to handle him, and remained introverted. However, she felt isolated and lonely in the church as she had no friends there. She later left the church and joined Living Faith Church in 2002, but the church was preaching prosperity gospel and she could not identify with the teaching, as there was no mention about the cross and the teachings of Jesus. She left and joined Victory Family Centre in 2003 to 2004, but did not join any cell group. She was contented where she was and attended church regularly, until 2005 when she joined Morning Star Church for a few months. From 2005 to 2006, she joined Alive Community Church and Tabernacle of Joy, of which later in 2007 she joined New Creation Church, Petra Church, Oikos Fellowship, 4 Square Church, Tabernacle of Fire; and in 2008 she joined South Asia International Fellowship. In 2011 she joined Koinonia Missions Church, and in 2012 to 2016 she worshipped at Cathedral of Glory. This church was very prophetic, and she received much learning during the sermons on Sunday. There was bible study on Thursday evening, and she grew spiritually. However, in 2016 she left the church as she could not fit in. From 2016 to present she worshiped at Cornerstone Community Church. This church is very vibrant in missions, as it is a mission's sending church. The church has over a hundred churches planted in the different parts of the world in Asia, Africa, Europe and the United States. She also has orphanages, schools and humanitarian projects all over the world. She has 6,000 members currently and is still growing daily.

Jill's Siblings

Jill has a third sister whom she constantly fought with. They grew up fighting. Jill appeared the stronger ones and would even hit her. They quarreled all the time and it was very miserable. One day Jill ran away from home and stayed at her cousin's new flat (as he has not moved in yet) with two of her classmates. Jill had a good time there, living like she had a holiday.

Jill has three brothers and three sisters, and she is fifth out of seven children. She did not have a pleasant time with her family in her growing up years, as each of them were individualistic and kept very much to themselves. It was only in her adulthood that she got more acquainted with her sisters and able to understand them better. Her eldest sister had gone home with the Lord as she passed away from bone cancer in 2016. Jill missed her, as they would have lunch often. They were close as they would go out often. She related with her second sister and third sister well now, although they had sibling rivalry when they were younger. Her three brothers were introverted, and their relationships were strained. Jill never knew them as their characters differed and they lived their own lives, very much separated.

Jill has been praying for her family's salvation for many years, as apart from her third sister and herself, the rest were all non-believers. Her mum, second sister and second brother were staunch Buddhist, but with God all things are possible. Jill believes that her whole family will be saved as Jesus is coming very soon.

Jill's Career

Jill left school when she was 18, as her first job was a Sales Assistant in a gift and jewellery shop. Her fond memories lingered, as she enjoyed her colleagues where she had good relationship with them. They would eat chicken pie often for tea-break. The owner of the jewellery shop had three other branches. He was a lucky man with three wives. The third wife would help to man the store. They would count the jewellery piece by piece each day and Jill enjoyed serving the customers.

After one year in the Sales Assistant job, Jill left and joined the Singapore Armed Forces. She signed a 5-year contract and her post was Technical Ordnance; where she handled the spare parts store for the army vehicles. During her 18 birthday, she had a car accident, as the car over-turned, and she broke her collar bone. She left the army after one year, as during the BMT, she asked for discharged because of the accident.

A life insurance agent who frequently came to her camp for business invited her to join him as a Life Insurance Agent. Jill joined Insurance Corporation of Singapore (ICS) as an insurance agent and was trying to pick up the business, but her colleague introduced her to a bullion company, which she later joined as an Investment Executive.

The bullion business was a very interesting career for Jill, as she traded in the futures market in gold trading. She had to look for investors to trade in the New York and Hong Kong markets. The New York market saw her marathon through the wee morning hours as it was day in New York and night in Singapore. She would go for early breakfast at about 4 am with her colleagues after the NY market closed. It was back to the office the next day at 11 am for the Hong Kong market. She enjoyed her work very much as she was exposed to futures trading in the bullion trade and got to trade for clients that she solicited. She would draw charts for minute-by-minute fluctuating prices in the exchange and read trends for the markets.

Jill was in the bullion business for about four years, of which later she heard a still small voice that nudged her to be a writer. She quit from her job and this was the beginning of her journey where she was thrust to an unending search to become a successful writer. She would write articles for magazines but she did not know how to build her career, as she had no guidance. She wrote her first article for a magazine but was rejected, but later she managed to write for Female, Sports magazine, Check-In, In Touch with the Family, Teenage, and did copy writing for companies.

Jill had a calling from God to be an evangelist in 1984, but she did not heed the call. Instead, she was hopping from one job to another. She knew that God has gifted her to be a writer, after all the bustle and hustle in wondering what she should do in the area of writing and ministry. In 1984, just at the same time she fell ill with schizophrenia, she received her call to be an evangelist. It was at this time that God began to arrest her spirit and taught her spiritual things. She learnt intimacy with God and to walk in His presence. God began to transform and change her thoroughly. She spent a lot of time waiting upon God, as He taught her persistence, patience, and tolerance. God taught her many things, and how to walk in the Spirit and not to gratify the desires of the flesh. Each mistake made was painful, as she learnt to listen to the voice of God and to walk in the Spirit.

Relationship with a Non-believer

Jill left church when she was 18, as she was involved in a relationship with a non-believer. When she was 15, she met James, a student at the Singapore Polytechnic. He was her pen pal when they met. Jill was in love, they would date weekly on nights and went to the East Coast beach. However, the relationship did not last, as after two years, they broke up. Nevertheless, when she was 17, they got back together and resumed their relationships.

"Jill, how do you like the beach? The waves are beautiful, isn't it?" James asked.

"Yes, the sound is so soothing."

"How do you like to come here weekly with me?"

"Oh yes, I would love to."

"Ok, set, we are going to grow romantically here."

"Yes, I like it. But promised me that I'll be back home by 9 pm. This is the curfew by my mother."

"No problem, baby."

However, after some time, their relationship took a turn as they began to quarrel almost daily.

"Can you cut the shit. I like to go home now." James added.

"But the night is still early. My mum wouldn't mind me coming home late."

"I am really tired, and I want to go home." James said.

"Why are you always in a hurry? Don't you love me?"

"Cut the crab. It is late."

They would hassle with each other when was the right time to go home, and they would drag their time until 2 am in the morning, and all they did was quarrel. This scene went on for quite some time, as they fought with each other and all hell broke loose. They fought incessantly, and Jill began to have nightmares almost daily. She would kick at the bed before she woke up in the morning, as she was distraught and deeply wounded. Life became hard for Jill as James would lie to her, hide things from her, but she would get violent with him and physically attack him. She would scratch him, and blood will flow from his hand, and their relationships was a total nightmare. This went on for many years. They kept their relationship for 9 years, from when Jill was 15 to 24 years. Finally, the day came, where they had to break up, and it was most miserable for Jill as she still could not get over him, still clinging to him, hoping for a miracle in the relationship.

There was a lot of pain in their relationships, as they were so different spiritually; Jill is a Christian and he is a Taoist. Their values and understanding of life were very different, as she would desire his love, but he did not really love her. They broke up in a very painful manner as Jill would hurt him emotionally, as all else went wrong. It was a big lesson for Jill that she should never get involved in a relationship with a non-believer again.

Life took on a new level, when the relationship Jill had, failed. Hopelessness, with despair, covered her in her inner most being. She had no purpose and direction. Her world collapsed before her, and daily Jill would spend time with God, to drown her sorrow and pain. Isolation became the norm for her, as God was her only refuge. The Lord taught her stillness and patience, and waiting upon Him. She would sit in her study room, and wait all day for God. It was through such a period that Jill grew to deepen her walk with God. She drew to God through intimacy with Him. Gradually she learnt to face the days with complete trust in God. The pain and heart ache changed the perspective as to how she handled her woes, and she had to learn to abandon her past. Life took on a new meaning, as Jill committed her total life to God.

PART 3

SCHIZOPHRENIA ATTACK

Jill finally went back to church at 24, when she left at 18. It was a time of healing of the soul, as Jill was badly wounded, after breaking up with her boyfriend and losing all interest in life. She couldn't care for her future, as she had no hope or aspiration in life. It was a life of denial, as she denied who she was, and took upon herself a lonely road to no where. Life was miserable for Jill, but she found strength in her faith in God. She began to trust Him for her healing, and four months passed, before finally Jill was sick with schizophrenia.

In a church camp in 1984, at Klang, Malaysia, Jill had her first attack of schizophrenia.

She drifted from her senses, and began to talk nonsensically. She walked around the camp site, and disrupted the meetings. A group of brothers-and-sisters-in-Christ had to pin her down to the floor, as she was violent and aggressive. She broke the window at one of the toilets, and the team had to send her back home. The next morning, one of the sisters-in-Christ packed her bag and a team of four brothers, with two at the front seat, and two others at the back seat, where Jill sat in the middle, and they drove her back home.

At home her mum attended to Jill after coming back from the camp. She slept for about a day or two; her mum placed sweet sour plum at her bedside, and after she awoke, she ate and felt good. However, she later left her house and roamed the streets. She performed signs to herself, talked to herself, played with a pool of dirty water, and attempted to throw herself to the oncoming cars. However, God protected her. She performed stunt by bending backwards and touching the ground. However, one of her former classmates spotted her and sent her home.

The next day, she manifested in her illness, as her family pinned her down to the floor and sent an ambulance that brought her to Woodbridge, a mental hospital. She was very sick and diagnosed to have acute psychosis. For two weeks she was bed-ridden. However, after two weeks she gained consciousness and was healed miraculously. Her church prayed for her and she recovered speedily. She stayed for another two weeks, after which she was later discharged.

First Relapse from Schizophrenia

Life was bitter sweet for Jill. Having fallen into schizophrenia, it was trying for her to receive her healing. The first relapse in 1989 saw Jill attending an International Missions Conference. Jill attended without knowing that she would manifest in mental attack beyond her control. She would walk and pace the floor, without knowing why she was doing so. She roamed aimlessly in the compound, only to see herself wandering without any purpose. She couldn't receive the teaching at the conference, but disrupted the meetings. She would go to the front stage, only to be brought outside of the auditorium by a group of ministers, who will coax and talk to her, to calm her down. Whatever the effort, Jill continued to be lost and confused. She talked to herself but couldn't relate with those around her. She couldn't identify where she was. There were so many sessions going on in the conference, but Jill just couldn't grasp as to what was going on. She had lost all sense of direction. The next day she would take a bus to the conference venue, but would miss the bus-stop and landed herself in another place.

However, at the conference, a minister would direct his gaze at Jill and seemed to communicate with her the Word of God, that through this conference, God had commissioned Jill to a full time calling as an evangelist. The minister prayed for her to fulfil her end time call, and Jill received it in the spirit. She left the conference, although sick, but with a commission to serve as an evangelist.

When Jill reached home, she had to content with her physical condition, as her family found her sick and sent her to the mental hospital. While at the hospital, Jill met all kinds of patients. Some were rowdy and very disturbed, shouting and yelling, while others were quiet and silent. Jill was particularly silent, as she kept to herself, didn't want to communicate and mind her own business. At times she would hallucinate and battle with the demons. She felt a strong sense of the demons harassing her, and she had to contend with it.

As Jill refused to take her medication, the punishment for her was injection. She would hide from the nurse for not taking her medicine, but was always found out. She learnt to adapt but didn't want to take her meals. She was forced to eat and it became an issue. They would send her to ICU ward where she would be fed through a tube that passed through her nose. She was fed with milk daily for an indefinite time until her discharged.

To Jill, her fasting was mistakenly seen as her refusal to eat her meals. She was fighting in the spiritual realm but the nurses couldn't understand her motive. The biggest struggle that she went through was during meal time, where the nurses would force her to eat. It was an agony that she had to learn to cope with. It was truly a nightmare for Jill, but however, she persevered and was able to get out of her predicament.

Second Relapse in 1992

It was at this time of Jill's life where she thought all went well, as she enrolled at Tung Ling Bible College and took the diploma course in 1992. She was doing well there, and went for a mission trip to Calcutta, India, at the end of the course. It was there at the trip that Jill fell ill as she could not take the toll of the difficult stresses there. While there, she manifested in sickness, where she spoke rubbish, pace about the floor unceasingly, and was very sick. She went there with Horizon Expedition, but had to come back as she could not take the pressure of the ministry trip. She was there for about a week, after which the team leader had to send her back, where she returned home on her own. Her family met her at the airport, and she was sent straight to Woodbridge Hospital.

While warded, she didn't want to take her medicine and had to be injected. She would spit off the medicine without the notice of the nurse but was caught and the painful punishment was injection. She was deceived that she was not sick and doesn't need medicine. Eventually she had to take the medicine as the nurses made sure that she took it.

It was at this time that God was so real to her, as she sensed His presence, as He talked and related with her. She would spend her time on her bed musing about God, as she watched through the window and sensed God in a powerful manner, as she looked into the trees and observed nature. The peace of God was so strong every day, that eventually she recovered quickly. She thanked God for His powerful presence, and it was because of Him that she was able to be discharged. Praise God for His goodness, as Jill will never forget His powerful leading in her life at the time of her most difficult moment. God broke through for her and she was so blessed with His mighty power and His awesome presence. He truly was a good heavenly Father. He healed Jill at the right appropriate time when she would be discharged and delivered from all her idiosyncrasies. He was truly the great heavenly Father who took care of her.

When she was down, it was God who cheered her up with victory. When the going looked tough, it was God who encouraged her. When things didn't go her way, it was God who strengthened her. She can do all things through Christ who strengthened her. (Phil 4:13). She can be confident of her God as He always sees her through in every situation, and He will not allow her to be moved. He knew and known Jill. He knew her struggles and setbacks. He knew her weaknesses and her need for Him daily. He never took His hand off her, and He was always by her side. Whatever that she was struggling, He will always lift her up no matter what happened. He was truly her Abba Father.

Third Relapse in 1996

The siren of the ambulance rang loudly, as Jill found herself kicking and shaking uncontrollably at the stretcher. Her hands were flying all over her head and her legs were stamping hard. Once again, Jill found herself at the familiar sight of the hospital bed. The stay at the mental hospital was trying. Lying at the bed, she would communicate in the spiritual realm, where she was contenting with the evil force that seemed to crouch at her. The evil spirits were battering with Jill, where she spent the rest of her stay at IMH fighting with them. The devil would echo through her ears, and it was a nightmare having to fight and resist the evil forces.

Jill would stare at the ceiling, and spend the rest of the time hallucinating and seemingly battling with the evil forces as they harassed and intimidated her. The nurse would push her bed away, and lead her to a solitary room, where Jill would fight with the devil.

After about two weeks, Jill would be up on her feet, rational and well. She would spend the rest of her stay there recuperating and gradually recovered.

She would then help in cleaning the cups and bowls, or sweep the floor. She made friends with the inmates and spent the time talking to them. There was not much that she could do except to watch television, work out some exercises in the morning, and do some creative craft that the nurses taught. It was very routine and mundane, yet it is the place to recuperate from her sickness. At times there would be some squabbles with the inmates, but she also made friends with some of them, as they would share about their own experiences and open themselves to each other about their struggles. It broke the boredom of the day when they could relate and identify with each other.

Watching television was a routine but at times the nurses would engage them in some activities like art and craft, where they did their drawings or played some games. Once in a while the male ward inmates would visit the female ward and they will have interactive time sharing and opening themselves to one another. At evening after dinner, they will stroll outside the ward, chatting and admiring the beautiful flowers. It was always good to chat with the male inmates as it was very therapeutic to communicate with them, as it helped in their healing.

Fourth Relapse in 2002

At the turn of the century, in 2002, Jill had her fourth relapsed. She had always thought that she was well and never to fall sick again, but this relapsed proved her wrong. She was expecting God to heal her, but she was very disappointed when she fell ill. There was always this spiritual battle that she was fighting whenever she fell ill. She was fighting with the demons and was attacked and struggled with the evil forces. It was always the battle with the evil one that she felt exhausted and spiritually challenged. God was always with her, but she had to fight this battle with gusto. Day in and out she could hear the devil speaking and tormenting her. It was a spiritual battle she had to fight to see God fulfilled His ministry for her. She was in God's training ground as she battled with the devil and learnt discernment in the spiritual realm. It was a war that she was constantly engaged in whenever she fell ill. It was a hard cold war, but she always won in God's sight. God would have her prepared for war before He launched her out to serve Him. It was a spiritual battle that she had to fight to learn spiritual understanding in the kind of war that she would be engaged in. God taught her and gave her spiritual insight on how to deal with the enemy. Ever since she first fell ill in 1984, she had always fought the similar battle – battling with the devil. The battle was difficult and hard, but she learnt to grow in this process. God was always by her side, and He aided her in every battle. The battle was always fought with spiritual lessons behind. Jill learnt to be dependent on God and trust Him for every move that she made. It was in times like this that she grew spiritually and relying on God for her victory. God always showed up and He was always with her. She learnt to abide in the Lord, and He directed and guided her path. (Prov 3:5-6). There were so many things to learn in the battlefield, and the most precious lesson was to be dependent on the Lord. Without Him she could do nothing as she made a lot of mistakes. She must give up on her self-identity and be connected with God to serve Him. It was always challenging to die to self and let God arise in her. She learnt to allow God to take charge in her life. It was difficult but necessary for God to train and use her. She must always rely on God in every area to see Him move on her behalf. It was heartening to realise that God was always by her side to help and train her, and she was always ready to receive a fresh move of God. With God anything was possible and without Him all things were naught. It was God by her side that allowed her to win all battles, even though it was hard and always trying. With God all things were possible and without Him all things would be impossible. She served a great God who was always with her, and He will never leave her nor forsake her. (Heb 13:5c). She can triumph as she hangs on to God and allows Him to do as He pleases with her life. With God she can conquer all terrains and see victory all the time. With God she can, and without Him she cannot.

It was during this period of difficult time that Jill grew in the Lord and allowed Him to teach her precious lessons. It was trying and yet necessary. Without the training she would not be able to rise and see God work in her life. The training was painful, but it was also very fulfilling. It was at this time that God broke through for her and she was healed.

Fifth Relapse in 2007

On 17th January to 10th February, 2007, Jill was warded at Institute of Mental Health (IMH) for her fifth relapsed. While she was at home on 17th January, two uniformed men came and wanted to bring Jill to the hospital. She didn't want to go with the men because she felt that she was not sick. They forced and tied her to the stretcher, as she struggled and tried to free herself.

For the first few weeks while she was at Ward 36B, it was a trying time for Jill. The nurses treated her badly and especially one Staff Nurse Ong, she was cruel and wicked and treated patients very badly. The Lord had assigned one nurse to Jill and she was nice and took care of her. As Jill resisted taking her meals, lunch and dinner were an agony as the nurses forced her to eat. She agonised through her month long stay but also learnt precious lessons to be patient and tolerant. Jill was transferred to the ICU ward as Jill didn't want to eat. She was warded alone in a room and spent time waiting and listening to the Lord. The waiting period was trying to Jill, as she was in solitary confinement without anyone to commune with.

The training from the Lord at the ICU ward was very trying, as the doctor supposed that Jill was not eating and needed feeding from the tube. However, staying alone at the ward was God's perfect place for her as He moulded and shaped her with His dealings. All her setbacks, hurts, and wounds were slowly dealt with by the Lord, as when it was time for her to be discharged, she had already received healing from the Lord in all her struggles and woundedness. It was healing time and restoration from the Lord.

Jill went through a process of cleansing and healing, as all her idiosyncrasies were dealt with. The Lord healed her from all fears and anxieties and woundedness of her spirit. Her spiritual walked with God at this time was the closest in all her life, as God met with her daily and healed her.

Daily Jill would watch the television, or she would spend intimate time with the Lord. She had so many questions, but didn't know how to relate it to the Lord. God will speak to her, and she would dialog with God. She spent her loneliness in the quiet presence of God, and God was so faithful to meet all her needs. She would bask in her fond memories to herself, as she shared with no one about her relationship with God. God broke through for her, and soon she was discharged.

Sixth Relapse in 2008

The sixth relapse that Jill had was between February to March 2008. Again, she was warded at the ICU ward, where she was alone by herself in a room. The ward was peaceful, and Jill spent the day hearing and waiting upon God, as she also encountered demonic activities, as the devil would speak and tried to confuse her. She learnt to listen to God's voice without the deception of the enemy, and it was a daily struggle discerning what was from the Lord and what was from the enemy. The presence of God allowed her to receive counsel from the Lord, and it was a marvellous time waiting upon

God daily. Day by day she experienced stillness and quietness, and it was the perfect ward to be in.

At the ward, she was fed with milk through a tube inserted through the nose; it was very uncomfortable and painful for her throat, as a hook was attached to the throat. She agonized day by day, always looking forward for the tube to be lifted. The day came when she was able to eat, and soon the agony with the tube was over. She was discharged as she ate her meals, and God healed her.

Prophetic Word – Exodus 23:20-23,25

The prophetic Word that the Lord had for Jill in 2008 was that God has assigned a Holy Angel to guard Jill in her path. He has prepared for her, to bring captives into His kingdom, where she has been sent to the enemy's territories to usurp the work of darkness and to bring many into His kingdom. However, she is to be on her guard with Him and obey the Holy Angel's voice and not be rebellious, lest He will not pardon her transgressions, for the Lord's Name is upon Him. She is to obey Him so that she will do what the Lord says, and He will be an enemy to her enemies, and an adversary to her adversaries. As she shall serve the Lord her God, He will bless her bread and water and will remove sickness from her midst.

The struggles that Jill went through with these other relapses in 2011/12, 2013/14, 2018/19 were the common traits of the constant struggle to cope with unreality. Jill found her answer in all the struggles in God. It was God who sustained her to cope with reality and to heal her; it was God who enabled her to fight the battles when her sickness was intense; it was God who gave her a hope to recovery in times of uncertainty; it was God by her side that enabled her to reach out to the other side of the rainbow when all else seemed grey; it was God who took her by her hand and lead her in the dark tunnel; it was God who gave her a hope and a future when all else seemed bleak; it was God who turned the situation around when all seemed hopeless. Jill found her significance in God as she clung on to Him who gave her a hope and a future. (Jer 29:11)

In all the relapses that Jill went through during the millennium attacks, she struggled but came through in the strength of God. The hopes that she depended was the Word of God. In Mark 11:22-24 – "Have faith in God. For assuredly I say to you, whoever says to this mountain, be removed and be cast into the sea, and does not doubt in his heart, but believes that those things he says will be done, he will have whatever he says. Therefore I say to you, whatever things you ask when you pray, believe that you receive them and you will have them." This were the very verses that Jill clang on when the situations seemed hopeless and in despair.

Seventh & Eighth Relapse in 2011/12

Jill, confining in the hospital bed in the solitary ward was most trying. She was all by herself, no one to talk to, in the silence of the day, where the only communication she had was with God. It was most boring with 24/7, but it taught Jill confidence in God and how to rely on Him. Each step in relating to God was most precious, as it was the only means to be occupied.

The time ticked away, hopes of discharge became grim, as Jill found herself engaging in fights with her inmates. Jill was watching her favourite television programme, when suddenly Mary came around and switch channel.

"Stop it!" Jill yelled. She went forward to change channel, but Mary lashed at her with a blow on her face. Jill retaliated and slapped Mary across her face. Soon a fight started and the nurses came running to the scene. The nurse pulled away Mary and Jill, and warned them to stop fighting. However, Mary shouted, "You idiot! Can I not watch what I want?"

Jill replied, "I watched this programme first. You have no right to switch channel."

The most profaning words came from Mary and they exchanged words in their disgust. The nurses charged them to be silent and switched off the television. Jill spent through the night sulking and in bad mood. She began to pray to God for her bad behaviour, and asked that she will never behave in that manner again.

The stay at the hospital can be boring. However, some craft work and activities brought life and vibrancy to Jill. The male ward was opposite the female ward, and they would at times visit the female ward and have some creative activities. The conversations with the two genders were very therapeutic, as they related and communicated with one another through the sharing in the discussion group. They would also participate in the morning exercises together, and it brought healing to the soul.

The stay at the ward taught Jill patience. She learnt to tolerate difficult situations with the inmates. She prayed to God and asked for strength. She began to reflect in her relationship with God, and desired greatly to be Christ-liked. Her confinement in the ward caused her to learn discipline and godliness. She desired greatly to be used by God to share the gospel with others. Her hope in God caused her to have hope in others. The least she could do was to pray. The condition in her surrounding made her feel despair. However, she knew that God was in control in everything, and that thought brought delight to her.

Nineth and Tenth Relapse in 2013 & 2014

It seemed that healing from mental illness was a non-reality for Jill, as year after year she had so many relapsed. Staying inside the ward was most boring, as time quickly flew by with the routine chore of breakfast at 8 am, lunch at 12 pm, tea-break at 3 pm, and dinner at 5.30 pm. Before an eye could blink, lights were switched on at 7 am and the patients were expected to take their showers. It took about an hour before all the inmates had taken their bath. Each stay was difficult for Jill, as there was no freedom to do what she liked, as the nurses kept a keen eye on the patients. Jill fought with the inmates before, and others too had fought among themselves. Some patients were intolerable as they made so much noise in their aggressions and disturbed the ward. It was most unbearable when the patients yelled loudly and shouting, destroying the peace.

Jill managed to make some friends there, and it made the day more tolerable as she could relate with the inmates. However, time passed by very quickly and in a twinkling of an eye she was discharged.

After her discharge, she will look forward to the day that she would be discharged permanently. There were many occasions where the enemy lied to her that she was healed. As Jill didn't know how to receive her healing, the years had dreaded to its ugly toll as she remained sick. Each time when she came back from her monthly doctor appointment, she would leave the hospital disappointed that she was not healed. She did not cry to the Lord for healing as she did not know how. She was not desperate enough to receive her healing and this was the reason why it took her such a long time to be healed. She learnt that God desired her to cry out to Him diligently and desperately, as He is the God who healed. As she did not learn her lesson, she remained sick for 37 years. It was a long struggle for Jill to receive her healing, but God remained faithful. He can heal and He will heal. It required Jill to cry out to Him with total humility and deep heart felt prayers that will touch God's heart.

Jill despaired with her condition, but God always hears the prayers of His children, and He has certainly heard Jill's cry. Glory to God. However, it was trying for Jill to hear God for her healing, as there was no answer because she failed to pray. It was a hard lesson that God only heals as He hears our prayers.

This relapsed was different from all other relapses that Jill had, because she couldn't hear God whether she was healed or not. At the end of her stay at IMH, she had to pretend to the doctor that she will take her medication when she reached home. She did not want to take the medication because of the last relapsed in 2008 where the Lord instructed her not to take the medication, but she took it and was not healed. She was convinced that she was healed and didn't need medication. However, all proved so wronged as the Lord directed her to take her medication. It was the toughest of her stay at IMH, as she never felt so lost and bewildered in all of her relapses. Instead of hearing from God, she skipped to take her own direction. It was very puzzling for her, as it seemed that God had abandoned her. She learnt a great lesson that she was not to disobey God and she needed to hear from God, as He was in control. It was a painful experienced, but God always broke through as she learnt to hear and yield to Him.

God was always in control but it was only through obedience that Jill could see the miraculous. It was always a miracle whenever God healed. Even though she had so many relapses, but she will always receive her healing in each episode. Each relapsed had its own experienced for Jill, but God was always the one who healed and set her free. Glory to God.

Final Relapse in 2018/9

God broke through in her final relapsed, as she went through 12 ECT in 2018 and 9 ECT in 2019. In both these years, her doctor saw to it that she was healed. After the treatment, she was completely well and could relate freely with people. She was exuberant, lively, and bubbling with excitement. Silence broke free as she was able to communicate.

In these two relapses, she lost her consciousness (not that she collapsed, but rather she didn't know her surrounding). She could not recall what happened to her, until the final two weeks prior to her discharged. Could this be the final healing after 37 years of fighting the illness? Jill praised God for His final healing as she has faith to believe that she is completely healed. He is the God who heals, and He is the God who saves. Jill was so thankful to a great and mighty God that she served. He is omnipotent and nothing can shake Him.

In 2018, Jill stayed at IMH from 1st October to 22nd November. It was a long stay. In 2019 she was admitted from 18th September to 6th November. Finally, after this last relapsed, God showed her four areas that she knew she was healed.

1) The deception of the devil was broken. In the past she had always have images that she was healed, yet she needed medication. As she looked through her journal diary, there were so many incidences that she believed she was healed but it turned out otherwise. The devil is the greatest deceiver, pounding on every opportunity to deceive and lie. As God healed, Jill began to see the tricks and lies of the enemy, and she begun to discern accurately what was of the devil and what was of God. It was a long journey, having stumbled along the way, but getting wiser each day.

2) She could read God's Word. In the past, she was always trying to understand the Word, but the Holy Spirit is slowly teaching her His Word and she found reading the bible more pleasurable than before.

3) She will allow God to lead her as she yields to Him. Waiting upon God can be difficult as she needed a lot of patience to hear God. Waiting upon God helped her to draw strength from Him as she persevered to hear Him.

4) Her character changed as she no longer had toxic thoughts. The enemy would put thoughts into her mind, and that was where she needed to

be resilient, to discern every thought that comes to her and to discard and resist the enemy when he puts toxic thoughts into her mind.

Jill can confidently trust God for her everyday living, without feeling helpless and hopeless, as she has aspiration and direction in life. She knew what to do every day and to live life to the fullest. God is great and she wants to serve Him with her fullest attention according to His perfect will every day. She desired to live life to the fullest, to find her destiny, and to fulfil her call as an evangelist, going to nations and preaching the Word of God.

Having received her healing, she can now serve God in her destiny, fulfilling all His will and doing great mighty exploits for Him. Life is like a flower, today splendidly displaying its beauty, but the next day it fades and dies off. Jill's life is in the hand of her creator God, as He leads and directs her path, and her future is bright. She serves a faithful God, and if He is for her, who can be against her. (Jer 33:3) – Call to Me, and I will answer you, and show you great and mighty things, which you do not know. Indeed, Jill's future is in God's hand, and nothing can snatch her out of His hand.

A Defining Moment in Jill's Life

Jill turned 61 and the defining moment in her life was when she was water baptised in 1985. She then enjoyed the new birth in Christ, and everything had its new beginning. Her walk with God was new; her relationship with people was new; life took on a new meaning as everything was new.

Being a child of God was special to Jill, as she began to know God and He imparted His love and grace into her life. She no longer was alone, and God helped and directed her path every day. She had new beginning and life took a turned from what was ugly to what was new and good. Her character changed, as she no longer was haughty and arrogant. Her bad temper went away, and she no longer kept to herself. She is a new creature in Christ.

Pastors Networking in Missions

In 2004, God instructed Jill to start a Pastors' Networking in Missions ministry. In lieu of Singapore being the Antioch of Asia, she was to co-ordinate a missions networking for pastors. The first meeting saw 10 pastors attending; where Pastor Matthew Teo from Bartley Christian Church graciously hosted the meeting at his church, and sponsored lunch for the pastors. The pastors will fellowship among themselves, and they helped each other network in world missions. Many pastors managed to network in the ministry and it lasted for about two years, after which later the ministry ceased because of poor attendance.

Jill wrote a book in 2001 about Singapore's Antioch call entitled The Call – The Challenge. It showed how the Singapore churches were fairing in world missions, whether Singapore has fulfilled the Antioch call and how churches were running with the Antioch vision.

She wrote the second book on the follow up of the Antioch call in 2014 entitled The Final Hour. It showed the pivotal final hour of the Antioch call, as it was critical that churches checked on how they have been fairing in fulfilling the Antioch call.

The destiny of Singapore being the Antioch of Asia was indeed a challenge to the churches here. Have churches finally fulfilled the call or was it still lagging in the air? They are responsible for their missions mandate, but it seemed that many churches are comfortable as to where they are, and it is just the minority churches that are active in missions. They are answerable to God for their actions and decisions. The Antioch call is to be embraced and churches must gear themselves for world evangelization. We are at the peak of our Lord's return, as Jesus is coming back very soon. Dare we hold ourselves from doing His perfect will? Dare we depart from the missions that God has entrusted to us?

Graduation from Asia Theological Center (ATC)

In 2016 Jill joined Asia Theological Center and graduated on November 1, 2020. The graduation service was on zoom, much to her disappointment. She got a Diploma in Missional Study. It took her four years of study there. Missions study was a very interesting subject. She enjoyed studying world missions and evangelism, and exposition of the New & Old Testament. Other subjects that she enjoyed were the Pentateuch, The Major and Minor Prophets, The Old Testament Survey, Bible Study Methods, Prayer and Inner Healing, and many more.

It was a time of refreshing course, and she was glad that all her classes were physical and not zoom, just before Covid 19 started in 2020.

A Prayer Answering God

In the midst of suffering and pain, God is the one who orchestrated everything in Jill's life. Through pain and sorrow, God can turn the tide around as He is Almighty God. Her struggle with mental illness taught her that in every situation, prayer is the only key to bring her closer to God and to receive her healing. She realised that through the many years when she was sick, she did not pray for healing and was complacent. It was a hard lesson but the reality was, God will not do anything if she doesn't pray. He is a prayer answering God. He desired that we turn to Him in desperate diligent prayer, as a means of our total dependence on Him. God will only move if we are connected to Him in earnest diligent prayer. Our destiny lies in our daily concerted prayers. Battles were fought with prayers. Healing took place because of prayers. Lives were transformed because of prayers. Miracles happened because of prayers. Our lives were changed because of prayers. If you want answered prayer, start praying.

Jill did not receive her healing any earlier because of lack of prayer. She knew no better that prayer was the key to her healing. However, God was kind and good to her. She experienced blessing and good health because He was faithful. In spite of her unfaithfulness to pray, He provided a path for her to walk intimately with Him. Every day Jill will wait upon the Lord for His dealings in her life. She would do nothing but simply waited upon the Lord. Each waiting drew her closer to God, as she began to understand His ways and dealings. We serve a faithful God who is faithful. His ways were not our ways and we could not fathom His ways. (Isa 55:8). He worked in ways that we cannot see, and we had to simply believed and trust in Him. There are too many questions we ask, but one thing remains constant, and that is God is who He is and we can simply trust Him.

Full Surrender to the Lord

In her lonely walk with the Lord, Jill discovered that God desired obedience in her. Doing His will was paramount to obeying Him. Every decision and direction that Jill made daily would mean dying to herself, with full surrender to Him. It was not easy to desire to do His will daily, as sometimes she went her own way and did what she wanted in her own strength. She was determined to walk with Him faithfully, obeying Him in every area of her life, and be willing to be directed by Him, in all that she does and be. It was a journey of wilderness for Jill throughout her waiting upon God for the last 37years. God wanted to perfect her, to totally surrender herself to Him, and to trust and obey Him. It was a lonely journey as she waited patiently for Him. However, one thing was true, and that was God had orchestrated everything in her life, to align her to His perfect will. Waiting upon God was a norm that became her habit daily. It was through waiting that she could perfect God's will in her life.

God had called out to Jill, to walk in His way and to partake of the fruits that He had for her. It was the fruits of the Spirit – love, joy, peace, patient, kindness, goodness, faithfulness, gentleness and self-control. (Gal 5:22-23). Perfecting herself in these fruits was not easy, as she tended to go her own way. God in His mercy, however, had provided a way for her, to walk in His way; by not losing sight of Him. It was through abiding that she could walk daily with God. He is faithful, and will remain so for as long as Jill walked and abided in Him. She served a faithful God and she can trust Him for everything in her journey with Him. He will never fail nor forsake her. She just had to cling on to Him and He will carry her in His everlasting arm. There was nothing that she needed that was without Him. He is always with her and He carried her daily. She is safe in the everlasting arm of her great and mighty God. His name is to be praised and He is truly a holy and faithful God. There is none like Him.

The Faithfulness of God

When Jill was sick, she only clung to the Lord. She did nothing but just sat at His feet daily. It was day after day waiting upon Him. Through it, it strengthened her walk with God as He became so real to her. She walked side by side with Him and communed with no one but Him alone. It was through this closeness that saw Jill through each time she fell ill. It was this intimacy that drew her to Him daily. It was through this time that Jill knew God was with her, and He was very real to her. Nothing beats the presence of God. He was close to Jill and His presence carried her through daily. In spite of the calamity when she fell ill, yet God was with her throughout her illness, and He proved to be the very present help in trouble. We served a faithful God and if He is for us, who can be against us. (Rm 8:31). No weapon formed against us shall prosper, and every tongue that rises against us in judgement we shall condemn; for this is the heritage of the servant of the Lord. (Isa 54:17).

One thing Jill needed, and that was the presence of God 24/7, in every minute and every moment of her life. It was in His presence that she could know Him and to be in His perfect will. God directed and guided her path. She needed to sense His presence daily and without Him she could not see the day beyond her. God is the heavenly Elohim; He was all she needed; and because of Jesus, she can face her tomorrow because He paid the full penalty for her sin. Jesus died that she might have the fullness of life. It was because of Him that she could live and breathe daily. He was the source of her strength and without Him she would still be steeped in her sin. Thank God for His Son Jesus who was willing to identify with us and died a cruel death for us. Because of what Jesus had done, we could now live with full assurance of our salvation in Him. We were once dead but now we are alive because of what Jesus has done for us. We could have this life salvation as we believe and accept Jesus into our lives. Our lives are whole because we have God and He is deep within her, as we soak in His presence daily. We have God because we surrendered our lives to Him. We can find and know God as we purposed in our hearts to know Him. We can find Him as we open our hearts to believe in Jesus. It is in Jesus that we can have abundant life. Jesus has already done all that He did on calvary cross. He died for our sins. He paid the full penalty for our sins, and when we believe in Him, we shall be saved.

Call upon Jesus while there is still time. God is on your side, and He will never leave you nor forsake you. (Heb 13:5c). He called and waited for you since time memorial. He is always waiting with open arms for you to acknowledge and accept Him. God has opened the way through Jesus. Trust in Jesus and you shall live life full of the peace and blessings of God. God loves you so much that He was willing to sacrifice His one and only Son Jesus for your sake. Because of us, Jesus was willing to go to the cross. He left heaven's riches to identify Himself with us. Call upon Him now and wait no more to receive Jesus into your life. God is waiting for you and He extends His arm to reach out to you. Wait no more to be saved. This is the day of your salvation.

PART 4

JILL'S JOURNAL

Finally, Jill would like to share with you her journal that she had collected through her journey. The years may not run in sequence. She had a collection of her years in memory, and she liked to share with you.

July 17, 2000
Doing Things God's Way

God had right from the beginning been telling me to abide in Him and do things His way. However, the flesh tended to disobey and I did what I wanted to do. This was the very essence of my mistake that caused me from fulfilling my ministry. Now I know clearly how I ought to do things God's way and not be yielded to the flesh any longer.

Please help me dear Lord Jesus to yield to you. Help me not to go my own way and do my own thing. Help me to obey You at all times and not grieve the Holy Spirit. Holy Spirit I ask that I will yield to You all the time and seek Your help in everything that I do. May You guide, lead and direct me. May You help me to follow Your instructions in everything that I do. Thank You Holy Spirit, thank You Lord!

Lord, I pray for your grace to help me through my relationship with my family members. May You grant me patience, love and forbearance for Your name's sake. Help me to carry out this task so that I will not grieve You with my character. Strengthen my weaknesses and grant me Your strength to grow in You. Strengthen my spirit man Lord I pray. Help me not to be weak but to be strong Oh Lord. Oh Jesus, thank You Jesus, thank You Lord.

July 26, 2006
Be the Best that I Can Be

This evening I was down, as I didn't feel like doing anything. I lazed and tried calling friends but the conversations did not satisfy me. I was as purposeless as ever and squandered my time away. However, God was good. He showed me that I must have an excellent spirit in everything I do. I prayed that I would be bubbly and energetic, full of enthusiasm and positiveness.

I also want to overcome the way I learn things and read. In the past, I just skipped and read through in my reading; but now I understand that I need to focus, grasp and understand what I read. I tried reading The Church Is Bigger Than You Think by Patrick Johnstone and I could read and understand it.

I want to have an excellent spirit, excelling in all that I do and be pleasing to my Heavenly Father. I want to focus in all that I do and I'll do well for God's glory.

Lord, please help me to be successful in everything that I do. Grant me an excellent spirit that I will excel in all that I do. Help me in my attitude that I will not be lazy. May I be found pleasing in Your sight, Oh Lord, my God and my redeemer.

July 29, 2006
My Birthday – To Be Transformed

God spoke while I was at Touch Heart Community Church, that I needed to seek Him and to pray constantly. I was convicted for not being diligent in my prayer life and I repented. God's Spirit was very strong at this Saturday's meeting at Touch Heart, as the theme was to Flow with the Wings of the Spirit of God. I thank God that once again He convicted me of my lack of diligence in prayer and I know now that in everything I do, and whatever I am believing God for, I must pray hard.

Dear Lord, I pray that I will pray hard in everything that I am believing in You for, that I'll be diligent to earnestly seek You. Help me to persistently pray for my needs and areas of my life that will glorify You. I thank You for the message this evening at Touch Heart by Bob Sjogrens about the cat and dog theology. I realise that I've been a cat, only praying for myself and asking You to bless me instead of praying that in every situation, Your name be glorified. Yes Lord, I want to glorify You in every circumstance of my life and I do not want to pray selfish prayer, of just blessing me. I want to pray that in everything I do, I'll glorify your name and lift You up and concentrate on You rather than on myself. I do not want to focus on myself anymore, but rather I want to pray that Your name be glorified. I pray that I will not ask for my problem with my family members to go away, but rather I want to pray that I will be strong to handle the situations and the circumstances with my family, and that I will be an overcomer. Thank You Jesus, thank You Lord!

Help me to focus on world evangelisation and see Your name glorified on the earth. May everything that I do glorify Your name. Make me an overcomer in every situation, so that I can handle the world and glorify Your name through what you want to do in my life. I dedicate myself to You once again and ask that I will honour You and serve You with reverent fear for who You are. Thank You Jesus, thank You Lord.

Aug 1, 2006
More God Centred & Less of Self

I read Larry Crabb's book, Finding God, that ministered to me. I realized that it was not I myself that was the center of my focus, but God. I had taken work as my top priority, instead of spending time with God. My relationship with God is all about Him. I do not live for my own pleasures, but I glorify God in my life. He should be the only reason why I did what I do. May I live to please Him.

Cat and Dog Theology

On Sat 29th July, I attended the church service at Touch Heart Community Church. The on-line video by Rev. Bob Sjogrens touched my heart with the message on dog and cat theology. The dog is one that will always run after the master and will jump and appreciate the owner with lots of licking and roll-over. However, cat just lies by itself and couldn't care less if the owner is around. It sits where it chooses and is totally oblivious of the owner.

The moral of the story is that the dog loves his master and would display its licking and jumping, whereas cat just simply ignores you. Bob pointed out that as the dog shows love by its licking, it says that the master must be god. The cat, which is always on the receiving end, could not care less about the master and therefore says that it (the cat) must be god.

In these two characteristics, we could liken our relationship with God, where one is hot and reached out to Him in love and adoration, whereas a cold Christian will just mumble prayers to suit their needs and expect God to meet their expectation.

I realise that I have been praying selfish prayer, with just my own needs being met. I do not want to focus on myself, but on God, and enjoy intimacy in His presence. I do not want to lead a pleasurable life without God being a part of me. God is the focus. I will gaze at God and tell Him that I love Him and I want to be diligently seeking Him. I want intimacy with Him and not take work as the priority.

In Genesis 4:8 we read that Cain murdered his brother Abel. He was punished by God for killing his brother, and became a fugitive and a wanderer (Gen 4:14). God said that he shall have no rest but a vagabond he shall be, traveling from place to place without a permanent home. Instead of repenting before God for his evil deed, he decided that he would build his own kingdom, by acquiring success as his means of survival. He was all for himself and tried to build his own kingdom. He had totally abandoned God.

We see Enoch in Gen 5:24 that he walked with God. His focus was on God and not on himself. God was the centre of his life and he communed and talked to God intimately.

I want to be like Enoch who walked with God and be found closed and intimate with God. I want to soak in His presence and seek him diligently and committing all my ways to Him. I want to know His character so that I can be like Him, holy and pure and pleasing to Him.

Dear Lord, I want an intimate relationship with You by seeking You and talking to You daily. I do not want to love work but to love You dearly. I commit all my ways to You and allow You to carry me wherever You want me to go and whatever You want me to do. I commit my work and ministry to You, and asked that You will be so real and close to me. Thank You for hearing my prayer as my desire is only for You. In Your most precious and holy name I pray. Amen!

The Lord also taught me to yield to Him in all circumstances. It came by yielding to Him and doing what the Holy Spirit said. I thank God that He is leading and directing me through each step of my way and He will deliver me from all harm and danger. I am thankful to God for the good times and the bad, knowing that I no longer lived for myself but for Him. I praised Him for vindicating me from the attack of the enemy and I can trust Him to deliver me from all situations and circumstances. Thank You Jesus, thank You Lord!

I tend to be angry when the enemy attack me, or with people that offend me. I relinquished my anger to Jesus and asked Him to remove anger off me and I will not be hostile when people wrong me. I want to yield to the Holy Spirit, and be full of love in dealing with people. I will to be gentle, assertive and not aggressive.

I praise God I am not alone, but He is with me to vindicate me. Glory hallelujah!

August 7, 2006
My Promised Land

I give thanks to God that I am healed from mental illness, as I have crystal clear mind to read and understand what I read. I thank Him for His healing touch and the long-awaited years trying to break-free from mental illness and to lead a normal life. I find myself breaking free from being work-oriented (whereby I chase after time to do my work) and now I am able to do my work, read God's Word without being pseudo-spiritual. Thank You Papa God.

God, I pray that I'll do well walking with You, never to lean on my own understanding again in everything I do. In every area of my life, help me to seek You and be utterly dependent on You for everything in my life. I want to be pleasing to You and I want an intimate relation with You where I can commune with You everywhere I am. I love You Lord and will not fall into the way-side or forsake or abandon You. Protect me from temptation and deliver me from the attack of the enemy, so that he cannot touch me. In Jesus most precious and holy name I pray. Amen!

August 8, 2006
Eve of National Day Celebration at Indoor Stadium

Love-Singapore celebrated National Day at the Indoor Stadium, and ushered in God's presence in Singapore. After many years of break since 2001, once again churches found themselves praying and crying out to God for revival. As I was at the Stadium, I wept. Simple reason that God loved us, but we had neglected our duty to bring about revival. We seemed to be disobedient towards our calling and missed the Antioch mandate.

We needed unity in churches, as our focus was on prayer. It was heartening to see so many churches coming together, to embrace the heart cry for revival. With 365 days and 52 weeks a year, one church can easily adopt a week of prayer for the next one year, with the other 91 churches participating. We stand strategically in the center of God's will, as we take block by block the HDB flats for the salvation of souls.

There were 3 points that we prayed for: 1) Prayer & Unity 2) Winning Singapore for Christ 3) Fulfilling the Antioch Call. It was encouraging to see us praying for Singapore and the nations. May we take Singapore for God and revival sprouting out in the land.

The end rendition at the stadium saw us worshipping God, as we sang that Our God is Great and We Serve an Awesome God (Our God is an Awesome God). I renew my covenant to serve God in the body of Christ, as we end the meeting with the Holy Communion.

August 10, 2006
Willing to Suffer for Jesus

Suffering for Christ is the last thing that one would engage in. However, Jesus suffered and commanded us to go through the same sufferings that He went through. It is through suffering that we will die to ourselves and take up our cross to follow Jesus (Lk 9:23). Every Christian ought to be willing to pay the price for suffering for Christ. Without which, it will be Christianity without power. It is required that we suffer, so that we can reign with Christ.

Lord, I am willing to suffer for You no matter what that cost. I want to make up with my family, and I want to go the extra mile to suffer so that I can win them over to myself and to You. Grant me the grace to go through whatever that You have for me and help me to be strong. Take away weepiness and let me rise up to every occasion. Help me to be the light that shines into the darkness and make me successful. Remove wrath and rage from me and help me not to be angry but to display Christlikeness.

Help me with my family situations, that I can talk to them and win them over. Helped me to be dependent on the Holy Spirit, and helped me not to lean in my own understanding. Helped me to handle my parents and siblings in the right manner so that Your name will be glorified.

Let my, This Little Light Shines for You so that I can bring You glory. In Jesus name I pray. Amen!

August 12, 2006
In Awe of God

Yesterday as I was spending time with God, I complained about having to consume haloperidol and fluanxol (my medicines), and blamed my doctor for having to take them, instead of cutting down the dosage. Immediately God's presence left me. I learnt that I must be holy and pure, ready for His used and not complain about my circumstances.

God also showed me my real character, as to who I am. I discovered that I am an introvert and tended to be childish towards God. God also spoke that I must make every effort to talk to my family members and make up with them for my bad relationship with them. I learnt that the only way for me to reconcile with my family members was for me to overcome them in their hostility towards me. I learnt to be confrontative, not afraid of my parents and siblings, and dared to challenge the devil in bringing strive between myself and my family. I wanted my true self to interact with my family members and not isolated from them.

I read today Nita Johnson's book The Breastplate of Righteousness, and was convinced that I needed to learn to study the scripture by praying over it. For example, if I come across the Word wisdom, I can claim from God this precious gift and pray over it to receive it from God. The book touched me with its writings on the garment, and breastplate of righteousness.

August 30, 2006
God, Restoring Me to Himself and My Love Letter to Him

I am at the beginning of my breakthrough from my past negative behavior. The Lord has restored me from a self-centered and carnal life, to one being able to walk with God in the Spirit and able to hear His voice.

I learnt to listen with my spirit-man, as this is where the Lord would speak to me, and not in my soulish realm. I made many mistakes in the past when listening to God, but I thank God that He will always see me through as I continued to yield and walk with Him. I am grateful for all the things that He has taught me, as I continue to walk in freedom and liberty in Him.

Thank You Jesus for changing my life and making me to what I am today. Thank You I no longer walk in carnality but in the Spirit of the living God. Thank You for pruning me and transforming me by Your power. Thank You for your grace to see me through with my past and thank You for Your patience with me. I am so grateful that though many times I failed to understand how I should walk with You, but You were ever so truthful and patient with me. Thank You Holy Spirit for prompting me to do what you want me to do, as I walk in the Spirit with You. Thank You Jesus, thank You Lord.

I loved You Papa God, Jesus and the Holy Spirit. Thank You I am covered with the blood of Jesus and the enemy cannot touch me. I thanked You for my calling to serve You in ministry, and I pray Lord that I will never look back for serving You. Give me joy that I once knew, that was robbed from me because of my disobedience towards you, in not giving heed to Your voice.

Lord, I am so grateful to You for restoring my life with You yet once again. You have outlined my ministry, as to what I will be doing until 2008. Thank You for straightening out my life with You before I operate in spiritual giftings and serve You in world missions. I look forward to it, in spite of the threat of the enemy that tries to discourage me from serving You. I thank You Lord I do not take heed of his blatant lie, and I know I shall enjoy serving You and the enemy cannot do anything to me. Thank You Jesus, thank You Lord. I loved you Lord for who You are to me. You are my loving Father who cares for me and wants the best for my future. Forgive me for my disobedience when I err from the truth. Thank You for forgiving me for all my sins. Thank You Jesus, thank you Lord.

This is the beginning of my journey with You oh Lord! May I do well to walk with you intimately, and to only hear from You and not do anything out of my own strength again. Thanked You for lifting me up from pseudo-spirituality, that I no longer be deceived by the enemy. May I walk with You in holiness, gentleness, purity, humility, pleasantness, and at the same time be strong and assertive and not weakening. Thank You Jesus, thank You Lord.

Jesus, I loved You. Thank You for being so patient with me. You have seen me through thick and thin – all the confusions You have seen it all. May I not walk in confusion anymore, but to walk in the Spirit with You and to always love You, honor You, and serve You. May Your name be the sweetest name, and may I love and yield to You all the time. Call me to yourself and set me apart to be used for your glory. Thank You Jesus, thank You Lord.

Holy Spirit, I thank You that You love me so much. You are so patient with me, that when I did not heed Your voice or to walk with You, You are still so faithful to see me through. Many times, I ignored You and failed to do what You said to me. I repent of my sins and ask You to forgive me for having quenched You and not walking with You. May I begin to walk with You in Your guidance, and may I yield to you all the time. Thank You Jesus, thank You Lord. Holy Spirit I LOVE YOU. Thank You Jesus, thank You Lord!

Thank You Lord for healing me of mental illness and arthritis, scoliosis, stomach condition, and my right ankle. I trust You to completely deliver me from all my infirmities. I trusted You to heal me and I give You thanks for all my healings. May I walk in intimacy with You, knowing You and serving You, and having faith to believe that my life is in your hand. In Jesus most precious and holy name I pray. Amen and amen!

July 29, 2007
My birthday – God asked me how I want my life to be

Today is my birthday. God asked me how I want my life to be. I told Him that I want to be a successful evangelist and a good and successful writer. I also ask for lots of friends and able to dine with many people at Sushi Restaurant, Korean barbeque, Thai food, Western food and so on … This is God's present for me. I turned 47 this year.

I now attend Petra Church, Rev John Koe being the Senior Pastor. Today is my second week. God also presented me with His gift, as He delivers me from the stronghold of dullness of the mind, sleepiness and mind-controlling spirit. He delivered me from the attack of the enemy and I thank God for His goodness.

August 9, 2007
Breakthrough in My Character

The enemy attacked me yesterday, with my mum accusing me for not throwing the rubbish. However, I was able to hold myself from anger, as I did not retaliate nor feel threatened when she scolded and attacked me. I was calm and steady, fully yielded to the Lord and only spoke when I needed to. The ice was broken, and the enemy defeated. I learnt that I would always go from the opposite reaction of the enemy, as that would neutralise the enemy's attack.

I felt total peace in the Lord as I yielded to Him and allowed Him to guide me in what I do. This is the breakthrough sign for me. In the past I did not feel good about myself, but for this week, I felt good and able to be energetic and enjoyed doing my work. This was the beginning of my victory. I thanked God that now I can make it with Him, and will serve Him with obedience and utter dependency on Him. Thanked You Jesus, thanked You Lord.

My Calling and Ministry
August 13, 2007

God is faithful even when I seem faithless. God, in His sovereignty, had given me talents, gifts and everything that I needed to serve Him. However, this problem of 'self' was always wanting to do things my own way. For 23 years, I fought the flesh and is still learning how to control myself. God had specifically showed me that I needed to abide in Him, draw close to Him, and not lean on my own understanding.

It was a painful thing to disobey God. It costs me everything, my ministry, relationship, work, and finances. However, I thank God that He is restoring myself to Him, and teaching me how to abide and yield to Him. May I be obedient to Him.

God has a call in my life. He called me to be an Evangelist and a Writer, spreading the gospel all over the world and being a good and prolific Writer. I am waiting upon God to teach me His Word and also to worship Him, and I am taking the whole month of August 2007 to edit and write, to master the craft of writing.

Come September, as the Lord led, I hope to take up writing courses and engage writing mentors. Hopefully

I'll write for magazines as I learn the trade of a Freelance Writer. *Lord, please help me to be successful as a Writer and Evangelist. Please show me what You want me to do every day, and lead me to the path of success. Bring people into my life that I can grow with, and prune my character so that l will have lots of friends. May you guide and show me what is success in Your guidance and leading.*

Lord, guide me every day to do your will without self-agenda but only Your plan for my life. Help me to make use of my time as You show me what to do every day. Let my days be smooth as I enjoy Your presence and guidance in my life. May everything be blissful and peaceful, full of Your love and grace.

God's Pruning Hand

Lord, please grant me Your grace to go through what You want me to go through. Help me to be pruned by You and be willing to yield to the Holy Spirit and do what the Holy Spirit says. Please help me to be obedient and to love You as You've commanded me. Give me the ability to love and help me to trust You that You will bring me out of the trial. Help me to co-operate with You and not do what the enemy says. I want to obey You and may I do well to serve and honor You.

Help me to be patient with people, and teach me to know how to handle them. Pave the way for me to serve You, and help me to be people oriented, loving them and be patient with them. Help me to carry myself well with people, and always abide and yield to the Holy Spirit, and only do what the Holy Spirit wants me to do. May I be yielded in Your hand and You direct and guide my path through each step. Thank You Jesus, thank You Lord!

August 14, 2007
Hurts and Pains

In 2 Tim 3:12, the Word of God said that if we desire to live a godly life, we shall be persecuted. Having a taste of what it meant, it challenged me to strive towards excellency in Christ, forsaking all self-effort and relying solely on the Holy Spirit's guidance and leading. I suffered in 2004 my mother's persecution. I was agitated and angry with her for the way she treated me, as she would side my siblings in our personal conflicts. When she attacked me, I would retaliate and shout at her. One day, as I was on my way to IMH for my monthly visit, the Lord spoke to me to be humble towards my mother. I didn't take heed, and thus the persecution in 2004, which lasted for about 2 years.

Today, I still suffer in her hand, as she still persecutes me and treats me with biasness. It pains me to see my own mother treating me in this way.

Lord, please take away the stress that I face with my mother. Help me to change in this process, and grant me Your grace to go through what You want me to go through. Help me not to be angry with my mother, and help me to forgive her for the way she treats me. Grant me favor with my family members, and help me to change in order to respond well toward them. Please take away all bitterness and anger that I displayed toward them, and help me to love them the way You want me to.

Dear Lord Jesus, please build up my character through Your Word. I love Your Word and I pray that You would teach me Your Word. Please come to me and teach me Your ways, and prune and groom me to be the person that You want me to be. Help me in my weaknesses, and strengthen me in all thy goodness. Grant me blessings and help me to serve my family well, so that all of them will come to know you. Thank You for their salvations and thank You for reconciling my relationships with my family members, as I give You thanks and praise. Thank You Jesus, thank You Lord!

As I suffer, it makes me strong. If not for my mother, I would not be able to control myself or remain Spirit-filled. The trials that I went through with her helped me to understand myself better, and to know that I needed to get rid of my baggage of hurts and anger that I never knew was residing in me.

Dear Lord Jesus, please take away the trial that I faced with my mother and help me to be her friend. I would very much like to help her in her response towards me, and I pray she would know You intimately and give her life to You. Help me not to quarrel with her but to give in to her. Take away my ego and pride and help me to be humbled. May You restore my relationship with her.

Jesus, grant me happiness with my family members and help me to have a lot of friends. Please guide my character and grant me mentors, peers and disciples. Help me to be discipled so that I can disciple others. Thank You Jesus, thank You Lord. Grant me favor with my church members at Petra Church, which I first attended in mid-July 2007. Please give me plenty of friends and that I'll be very successful serving You in helping to change lives. Give me the skill that I need to handle people, and grant that l will know how to handle relationships and overcome the enemy in Jesus Name.

Whatever the enemy has done against me with my family members, undo it oh Lord I pray. Grant me good relationship with my family members and enable me to relate and talk to them. Grant me favor in Your eyes, that they will treat me well as I surrender all my responses towards them to You. Help me to be polite and not rude, to be nice to them. Grant me wisdom to know how to treat people, so that I can fulfil my high-calling by being a friend to others. Removed anger completely from me, as I still have anger within me. Grant me a pure heart that I will not have evil thoughts in my mind, as I belong to You and You manifest in me. Thank You Jesus, thank You Lord.

Help me to fulfil my destiny in You oh Lord. Make me a prayer warrior and to take cities for You. Gear and prepare me for world evangelization. I want to see nations giving their hearts to You and the gospel travel far and wide. Help me to be ready to serve You. Equip me with Your Word and to fellowship with my spiritual family. See me grow in my faith in You and help me to always please You. In Jesus name I pray. Amen!

August 27, 2007
My Dreams & Aspirations

The best dream that I can ever have was to fulfil the dreams that God gave me. There is no other pleasure or delight than to know that I am doing God's will and pleasing Him daily. My aspiration is to do God's will and to please Him in every area of my life. I want to love my God as I should, and I thank Him for continuingly shaping and molding me into His image. I want to have the character of Jesus, and I want Him to reign supreme in my life. There is no purpose and goal in life than to be serving God. Serving Him is a pleasure and I want to commit all my ways to Him, through prayer and intercession and not lean in my own understanding.

I am gifted with the talent to write. I want to excel in this area. I want to free-write every day, take up courses on writing and do well. I want my talents to grow and I want to serve Him in His terms and not mine. I submit to Jesus, His Lordship over my life, and I abide and yield to Him every second and every moment of my life. *I love You Lord!*

God had so graciously called me to be an Evangelist and an Author of books. I want to serve Him whole-heartedly in these areas and I want to have an excellent spirit to serve Him well. I want to be able to handle people from whatever levels they may be at and not be ashamed or inferior toward them. I fear no one, and I submit my ways to the Lord and only feared Him alone. No humans and no demons can swirl me otherwise, as I have the Holy Spirit, and He will protect me from danger and harm, and I totally and completely submit to Jesus as my Lord and Master. *I love you, Jesus!*

God has given me the covenant to serve people. I am to touch lives, heal the sick and cast out demons. I have the mind of Christ and I want to operate in full authority in the Lord. I want to serve people well, and I want to be able to handle relationships at all level. I want to be people savvy, I want to love the unlovable, and I want to be patient with people who are under bondage to the enemy, and I want to help them with the guidance of the Holy Spirit. I want to serve people the way that the Lord wants me to. May He help me to do well and know how to handle people and the enemy. I want to be so skillful in handling people, that the enemy's plots and plans against me will be taunted.

I want to be a great Evangelist, preaching God's Word and sharing the gospel to see lives touched and changed by the power of the living God. I am a world Evangelist, preaching the Word all over the world, beginning with my family right now. I chose patient rather than rage and anger, and I chose to treat my parents and my siblings well with the right attitude toward them and show them my love. I want to yield to the Holy Spirit, and allow Him to guide and direct my path with my family members. May I be a blessing to my family members and to the world.

I want to be a great Writer, writing books that will bless many, and help them to walk with Jesus. I want Jesus to be magnified and His Name glorified. In every book that I write, I want to be guided by Jesus, that in everything I do, I am directed and guided by the Holy Spirit. *I love You, Holy Spirit.* I want to write many different types of books that will bless people. May Jesus teach me the ways of Him and help me to help others.

October 3, 2007
Singapore@Prayer - Prophetic Word

Tonight at Singapore@Prayer, the Lord moved prophetically with His Word in Isaiah 1:24-26 –24Therefore the Lord God of hosts, The Mighty One of Israel declares, "Ah, I will be relieved of My Adversaries, and avenge Myself on My foes." 25"I will also turn My hand against you, And will smelt away your dross as with lyre, And will remove all your alloy." 26"Then I will restore your judges as at the first, and your counsellors as at the beginning; After that you will be called the city of righteousness, A faithful city."

I thank you Lord, for Your prophetic Word. Thank You for telling me that You will smite all my enemies, and You alone will do it. Thank You! You would also lift up all my dross, all my filthy behaviors, every anger, rage, wrath, hostilities, frustrations, and every behavior that displeased You. Thank You for telling me that I will judge myself, so that I will not be judged by You. I repent of every behavior that was full of rage and anger. I ask You Lord to completely remove it from me. Thank You Jesus, thank You Lord!

Finally, you will restore me to the body of Christ, where I would have Spiritual fathers and Spiritual mothers, with pastors and leaders overseeing me. I would never be alone again, for I will be surrounded with the Spiritual family that will bring me much joy and happiness, as I serve You in Your Kingdom. Thank You Jesus, thank You Lord!

These prophetic Words, were the Word of the Lord for me. I received it, and would embrace every Word that was spoken to me. I was so glad and grateful that the Lord will fight my enemies for me, and He will restore me to Himself. All my dross, alloys, and ugliness will be removed. Finally, He will give me a Spiritual family that I have been crying out to Him for.

Lord, I thank You for healing me after all these years of praying. It was a very long time praying for healing. I thank You that the spirit of doubt and unbelief was cast out, as he attacked my faith about being healed. Please forgive me for not being diligent in prayer. I prayed everyday but without intensity. You want me to earnestly cry out to You, and I would do as You said. Thank You for healing me as I truly appreciate it. I loved You Lord and I wanted to obey You in everything that You said to me, and I want to serve You wholeheartedly and pleased You in every area of my life. May I be found faithful to serve You well and be a great Evangelist for Your glory. Helped me to do well and not be in the fresh, but to be in the Spirit all the time.

Help me to be yielded to You, and to abide in You, and carry Your presence. Help me to be sensitive to abide in you and not to be distracted by the enemy or be swayed by him. May I do well in everything that I do and Your name be magnified and glorified. I want to walk closely with You and I want to linger in Your presence all day long. Help me to think of You all the time. Once again, thank You for healing me and I love You so very dearly oh my Lord. Amen!

I realised that I had been hostile and aggressive towards those who wronged me. Lord, I want to develop my character by being humble and not hostile. I do not want to hate anti-Christ person, as I want to handle them the way You want me to handle. Help me not to hate them. Thank You Jesus, thank You Lord!

I want to build my relationship with my family, and I want to pray for them regularly. Help me Lord to talk to them and not keep to myself. Liberate me that I can talk to my family members. Change and transform me oh Lord. Help me to build relationships and know how to handle people.

November 3, 2007

This afternoon as I was in God's presence, I began to weep and pray for myself, as I was doing things my way. Many times, I disobeyed God by going my own way but He would gently nudge me and bring me to Himself. But this afternoon, I wept and felt sorry for my attitude and sin of independence. Thereafter I could hear God clearly and able to discern the attack of the enemy with clarity and sharpness. I began to enjoy waiting upon God as I overcame all deception and attack of the enemy. *I am so grateful oh Lord for having been kind, tolerant and patient with me all these years when I failed to yield to You. Thank You for showing me Rm 2:4 that said, "Or do you think lightly of the riches of His kindness and forbearance and patience, not knowing that the kindness of God leads you to repentance?"*

Thank you, Lord, for being so kind to me, picking me up each time I fell. I am so grateful that You were always with me, never to leave me nor forsake me. Thank You for the breakthrough to hear from You clearly and not made mistakes. Thank You Jesus, thank You Lord.

May I walk humbly with You, pleasing You in every area and be abiding and yielding to You always. Thank You I am a new creation in Christ; my old has passed away, behold the new has come. (2 Cor 5:17). Thank You Jesus, thank You Lord.

November 6, 2007
Gift of Healing Released

The Lord was so good. I received my breakthrough in ministry when the Lord graciously gave me the ministry to heal the sick. This word was released by Karen Dunham at Cornerstone's church meeting. In the meeting, the pastors and leaders formed a chain of tunnel for the participants to go through and to pray for them. Rupert prayed over me with the anointing, as I felt the anointing of the Spirit of the Lord flowing through me. Then a lady of about 60 years (supposed she's an American) jokingly said to me that the Lord will use me in spite of my weaknesses. Then Michael Ross Watson sang over me with this word – "the arm of flesh will fail you and you dare not trust your own." Finally, Karen Dunham prophesied over me that the devil is defeated in my life and they can do nothing to me. Finally, she said that the Lord has given me the gift to heal the sick. I want to make use of this gift to pray for people, as I want to be a good steward of my gift. I want to pray for my mother's both knees to be healed and her insomnia healed too. Thank You Jesus, thank You Lord.

While walking through the tunnel, I felt the enemy getting hold of me through a lady that prayed against me from the back. As I went back to my seat, I figured out what that would really mean, what the enemy would hold against me. I ask the Lord what does that mean, and I found myself praying in the Spirit, with one of my hands raised high and my second finger pointing to the air, and I was shouting out loud to the devil to take his hand off me; that he cannot hold me anymore. Thank God the demon left me, and I was completely set free. Wonderful Jesus, wonderful Lord.

I came back from the meeting truly blessed of the Lord, and I checked Galatians 5:16 with this word – "walk by the Spirit and you will not carry out the desire of the flesh."

Dear Lord Jesus, I love you. Thank You for loving me and taking care of me. Thank You for your provision for my needs, as there is no lack. Thank You for the food on the table, clothes to wear and a roof over my head. Thank You for the breakthrough in the spiritual realm, that I can serve you in the ministry of healing. I arise with complete peace as I soak in prayer in His mighty presence.

Lord, please heal me of my memory, that I can remember things and also to grasp information clearly. Lord, You asked me what did I get out of the message from Karen Dunham's meeting, and the answer was that I had completely forgotten what was shared. Lord, I pray that You will help me to remember things and that I will have a crystal-clear mind to grasp sermons, and able to understand lectures, able to read with understanding with the Bible; and also reading my books and magazines, and everything that I set my hand to read. Thank You Jesus, thank You Lord.

November 8, 2007
Breakthrough for my Spiritual Walk

Today was special because I saw things clearly without deception. On Tuesday night (Nov 6) after coming back from Karen Dunham's meeting at Cornerstone Community Church, I was completely lifted in the Spirit. However, the enemy began to strike me with pseudo-spirituality. I began to wonder what I should do, confusing me and attacking me with deception. I got up the next morning completely out of touch with God, as I was under attack. I managed to get out of it by taking authority in Jesus' name. The enemy was subtle as he tried to attack my high moments with the valley.

I thanked God for what He is doing and will continue to do in my life. I was completely thankful to the Lord for His great mercy in seeing me through. *Lord, I love You. I want to tell You that I am so thankful for the things that You teach me regarding ministry. I thank You that You are faithful to do what You said You would do. Thank You Jesus, thank You Lord. Thank You for healing me of mental illness that I can see things clearly and be delivered. Thank You for your promises, and I look forward to my victory.*

November 12. 2007
Cross Over – Yielded and Abiding in the Lord

Devotion – Jer 31:13-14 – [13]"Then the virgin shall rejoice in the dance, and the young men and the old, together. For I will turn their mourning into joy, and will comfort them, and give them joy for their sorrow. [14]And I will fill the soul of the priests with abundance. And My people shall be satisfied with My goodness," declares the Lord.

This morning during my quiet time, the Lord referred me to Jer 31:13-14. I have gone through much pain and trials with my family members these past years, that my communication with them is affected. I thanked God that the enemy cannot attack my relationship with my family, as the Lord said I shall rejoice in the dance, and He shall turn my mourning into joy and He shall comfort me. He will also fill my soul with abundance. He shall satisfy me with His goodness and all that He has for me is very good indeed.

The Lord shall bless my coming in and my going out, and He shall fill my broken cistern with water. My belly shall be filled with the rivers of the living water as the Holy Spirit fills me to the over brink. The Lord is my joy and my strength. He shall be my delight and I shall be a special treasure to Him. (Exo 19:5). Thank You Jesus, thank You Lord!

For the last two days I had been attacked from my computer with the letter 5 appearing. The Lord taught me spiritual warfare, as He showed me how not to be angry, but to handle the enemy assertively. This morning, again, my computer was under attack, and the Lord told me not to be stressful. The best way to handle the enemy was to be assertive, silent, and not be angry, and to take authority. I could take authority without getting angry. *Thank You Lord for teaching me how to handle the enemy. Thank You Lord I am no longer an angry person, but Your daughter filled with love, patient, kindness, goodness, faithfulness, gentleness, self-control, with joy and peace filling me all over. Thank You Jesus, thank You Lord! Thank You all anger had melted away, and I thank You that I am no longer angry with my family members, for the way they treated me, but I will exercise assertiveness in handling them. Thank You anger is gone, and assertiveness and confidence will be my stay. Thank You Jesus, thank You Lord.*

I had crossed the line over, where I no longer do what I want to do on my own strength, but I commit my work to the Lord. I do only what He wants me to do and I acknowledged His sovereignty over my life. I will yield to the Lord and commit all my ways to Him. I am able to read God's Word, as my mental mind is healed and I obey the Lord as to what He wants me to do. May the Lord see me through as I continue to abide in Him, draw close to Him, and allow Him to manifest all His ways in me. *I loved You Papa God; I loved You Jesus and the Holy Spirit. Amen.*

November 15, 2007
A Memorable Day – The last day the devil is going to lie to me.

Today is the last day that the devil is going to lie to me. Lord, I seal it in my prayer to You Lord. The devil seemed to get away with his lies by asking me to stop reading God's Word, go and take my dinner, speaking to me externally to do things. I will not be deceived by him anymore, because God spoke to me from within and not from without. *Lord, I learnt to discern against the deception of the enemy, Lord, and I will not fall into his deception to do anything that the enemy asked me. I am determined to walk out of deception, resist temptations, and do well by doing what You said by engaging my inner man. Thank You Lord I will not be deceived and I*

overcome him by the blood of the lamb. Thank You Jesus,
thank You Lord. Amen!

November 26, 2007
Doing Things with Self Effort

The Lord was so good. His mercy endureth forever.
Recently I got my breakthrough but I doggedly wanted
to read God's Word without abiding in Him. The
reading was dry and frustrating, as I could not grasp
what I was reading. Finally, the Lord revealed that once
again I had done things in my own effort. I repented
and began to discern not to go my own way. Praise the
Lord!

The Lord revealed to me yesterday about the tasks I
did which were not covered in prayer. I did what came
to my mind without praying and discerning. I realised
that without discernment the enemy would relentlessly
attack with deception. He would urge me to read
God's Word, to hinder me from truly understanding
the Word. Reading the Word became stale and boring.
Thanked God, He was always in control, and He will
reveal the truth to His children.

December 9, 2007
Conviction of my character

The Lord gave me the Word in Isaiah 43 that He
loves me and I need not fear anything. Glory be to God.

Verse 18 says, "Do not call in mind the former things, or ponder things of the past. Verse 19 - Behold, I will do something new, now it will spring forth. Will you not be aware of it? I will even make a roadway in the wilderness, rivers in the desert." These verses speak to me about my restoration with my family members; that my pasts are over and done with, and behold, now, I am a new creation in Christ. This verse also speaks about my wilderness, that it will end soon, as the Lord will pave the way for me with rivers in the desert.

I need not walk in the past, as the Lord is doing a new thing in my life and I shall receive it in Jesus' name. All the hurts and wounds with my family members were healed and I shall call my wall salvation and my gates praise. Praise the Lord! *Dear Lord Jesus, I thank you that my relationship with my family members is healed, and I can walk through my wilderness period with victory. Thank You for making a roadway in the wilderness for me, and streams of rivers in the desert. Thank You Jesus, thank You Lord. Amen!*

January 31, 2009
Structural Weakness

Weakness – the core of my characteristic that prevented me from serving the living God any earlier. The Lord revealed tonight that I have a structural weakness that caused me from advancing in serving Him. I would always please people, and will do anything to please them. Even if people were to violate my space, I would still rigidly go along with their attack in my life. I allowed people to tell me what to do and I would relentlessly give in to them. This 'giving in' to people caused me to be weak, and refrain from making my stand with people.

Dear Lord Jesus, thank you for arresting my weaknesses and causing me to deal with it. Thank you for showing me my tendency to please men and the fear to offend them. Thank You Jesus for strengthening me now and giving me a hope to serve You in spite of my weaknesses. Thank You I can now handle my family with tact, no longer weak but strong to handle them. Thank You Jesus, thank You Lord!

Now I am ready to write and run with my writing ministry and my full-time calling. I will write articles and books and to have favour with men. I will run with the vision and I will be strong and mighty, able to handle people well without pleasing them. I will be bold with people and rise up to handle them well. I look forward to my new lease of life and will eagerly wait upon Jesus to lead and direct my life. I will wait upon Him, commune with Him and not go my own way. I know how to live without getting pseudo-spiritual. May Jesus be my guide and strength. Amen!

April 15, 2009
Breakthrough

The Lord met me in a tangible manner as I surrendered my all to serve God. I felt that all past inhabitation with my family members has been lifted up. I found new purpose and direction, able to know what I needed to be doing, and be victorious in Jesus by knowing how to handle my mother and my family. My relationship with my third sister had always been a mire, as we fought since young, even up till now, as we only talk when necessary. I pray for good relationship with her and I know God will answer my prayer.

My countenance has changed, as I know how to handle people appropriately. My breakthrough is at hand, as I no longer fear men, but is courageous to handle them without inhabitation. I sensed God healing me and making me whole again. All my past hurts and wounds have been healed in Jesus' name. Glory hallelujah.

May 29, 2009
Lifted up from the spirit of rejection

As my relationship with my third sister is passive and I cannot relate to her, the Lord shows me tonight that it is because of the spirit of rejection that I am unable to communicate. The Lord sets me free tonight as the spirit of rejection is lifted up from me. The Lord has revealed that as I'm set free from rejection, I'll be able to relate with my family freely. Glory and praise to Papa God and Jesus and the Holy Spirit for healing me of rejection. Jesus whispered into my ears with this word – "I love you". It is the most soothing word that I can hear from the Lord. Thank You Jesus!

June 29, 2009
Must gear up for Spiritual Warfare

Time flies, real fast. Just a twinkle of an eye it is now the end of June. What have I accomplished for the past six months then? Preparation. Character development and moulding by Jesus. The flesh was in the way of the Lord; therefore, I learnt to walk in the Spirit. Yielding to Jesus is the key. Being utterly dependent on Him is the right way to walk with Him.

The Lord revealed my structural weakness in January, and how much have I changed or grown in? How much do I spend time praying and crying out to God regarding my situations? I cannot continue to be passive. I need to rise up. I must not fear or please men, and I must be myself, confident and positive.

Help me Lord to be positive and confident with myself. Grant me relationship and help me to know how to relate to people. Give me the gift of the gap to communicate, oh Lord I pray. Thank you for answering my prayer oh Lord.

Lord, I must rise up. I want to fulfil my destiny in You. The ministry you have given to me is wonderful. May I pray like never before and see breakthrough for myself, my family, and ministry. May I be yield to the Spirit of the living God to help me. Amen!

July 3, 2009
Being Yielded to Jesus

I found that when I didn't plan my time for the day, I can be aimless. However, Jesus taught me to plan my work so that I can be fruitful for the day. When I do plan, I have purpose as to what God wants me to do. I am not aimless but I strive to serve Jesus at His command, as He guides and directs my path daily. I want to yield to Jesus by acknowledging Him in all that I do, so that I will have an intimate relationship with Him.

Jesus, I ask that I may be in Your presence all the time, seeking and yielding to You. Help me to abide in You closely, so that I will not lose sight of You. In Jesus' most precious and glorious name I pray, amen!

July 5, 2009
May we be liked Moses – (Exo 3:11-15)

There are 5 things that we need to take note of, just as Moses struggled in all these 5 areas.

1. Who am I Lord? – We see our own inadequacy and question ourselves in our ability. God's

answer to us is that He is sufficient in us, and as we are being led by Him, He can help us in our destiny.

2. Who are you Lord? – We struggle in our own intimacy with God by not knowing Him, but God says He is the I Am, and we are to trust in Him.

3. Lord, I am not good enough – we struggle in intimidation as others try to pull us down.

4. Lord, I can't speak – we struggle in our own inadequacy and look within ourselves, at our own limitations.

5. Finally, we say, send someone else Lord – we feel that we can't make it and suffers inferiority complex.

We are to trust God with our calling, and we need to honour God with the giftings that He gives us. We must rise up and fulfil our destiny. We can only succeed when we look to God solely. Like Moses, we have our own idiosyncrasies, but we are to trust God in all our circumstances. We can be the pillar by standing on the promises of God, and believe that in Him we are all sufficient.

August 28, 2009
Persistency, faith and resistance

The Lord taught me today to learn to persevere in prayer and not pray whippy prayers. *Lord, I pray that*

You will forgive me for not praying from my heart strong prayers and mountain-moving type of prayers. Thank You for showing me my prayer condition, that I do not pray for healing for all my infirmities. I realise that I did not cry out to you intimately for my conditions, and I ask You Lord to forgive me. Lord, I need to pray for my father, mother, and my sibling's salvations. Grant that I will pray for them daily and with earnest prayers. I also pray for my work – writing, that I'll do well in my career and be financially blessed. I need to look up to You and be utterly dependent on You for everything. Help me to cry out to You diligently and receive all my breakthroughs. Thank You Jesus, thank You Lord.

The second thing that the Lord showed me is that I needed to be resistant to the enemy's attack. The enemy attempted to attack me with clutter mind but I resisted him and he fled from me. I learnt the power of resistance, as I do that, the enemy cannot touch me. *Thank You Lord that the enemy cannot attack me with mental illness attack and distress and clutter attack. He has to depart from me in Jesus' mighty name and never to attack me again. Amen!*

The third thing the Lord taught me is not to believe the doubt of the enemy. Faith needs to arise and not believed the enemy. *Lord Jesus, thank You for mountain-moving faith and not have doubt and unbelief in me. Sorry for the past that I tend to doubt your promises, but now I choose to believe your goodness and your blessings. I choose to believe that I am already healed from all my sicknesses, as by Your stripes I am healed. Thank You for the manifested healing that takes place in my body. Thank You Jesus, thank You Lord.*

My memory is healed in Jesus' name, as I receive healing for my mental mind. My brain cells are normal and contain genius cells and wisdom cells. I am thankful for wisdom and character, that God gave so lavishly.

Thank You Lord that I am healed in Jesus' name. There are no sicknesses that can come upon my body as I am covered by the blood of Jesus. I am whole and complete, and I have a sound mind to relate and reason with people. All my hurts and wounds are healed in Jesus' glorious name. Thank You Jesus, thank You Lord!

November 21, 2009
Thankfulness Towards God

I am thankful towards God for His goodness and faithfulness. He showed His love by teaching me obedience. I was so grateful for His abounding love, that He loved me unconditionally in spite of my sins. I would look to Him for everything that He was to me.

Papa God, grant me wisdom and discernment to serve You. Protect me from the evil one and grant me favour with men. Show me Your unending love and thank you for my family's salvation. Grant me good relationships with my parents and my siblings. Thank you for a successful ministry as a writer. Help me to write prolifically and to be a good writer. Help me to craft well written articles. Thank you for Your anointing to serve You. May I be yielded to You and be utterly dependent on You always. Thank You for the new lease of life that I found in You. Thank You for character and the power to serve You. I look forward to my ministry and breakthrough to come forth in my life. Thank You Jesus, thank You Lord. Amen!

December 6, 2009
Prayer for Guidance

God was always with me. He constantly guided and protected me. He was my shield and defender. He directed and led me in the path of righteousness. He is my delight, and I shall rest in His guidance. I serve a God who cares and knows me. My life is in His hand. He will carry me in all life's struggles and He will be my constant guide. I am so glad that I serve a good and faithful God. I am forever thankful and grateful to Him. He is all that I have. Glory to God!

I want to serve You oh Lord, that I will carry your presence and peace wherever I go. I want to obey You, commune with You all the time, and be yielded to You every moment and every second of my life. Helped me not to lose sight of You but to always abide in You and feel your guidance and leading. This is my sincere prayer to You oh Lord, asking You that You will answer my prayer and see me through my relationship with You. In Jesus most precious and holy name I pray, amen!

Now I am ready to write and run with my writing ministry and my full-time calling. I will write articles and books and to have favour with men. I will run with the vision and I will be strong and mighty, able to handle people well without pleasing them. I will be bold with people and rise up to handle them well. I look forward to my new lease of life and will eagerly wait upon Jesus to lead and direct my life. I'll wait upon Him, commune with Him and not go my own way. I know how to live without getting pseudo-spiritual. May Jesus be my guide and strength. Amen!

March 27, 2010
Creative Miracle

I experienced a creative miracle from God today when I had my dinner. There were only two pieces of sweet-potato with the porridge in it; but when I was eating, I realised that there were so many pieces of sweet-potato. It was a creative miracle from God. This is the first creative miracle that happened to me. Praise God. *Dear Lord, thank you for the many pieces of sweet-potato that you provided for me during my dinner tonight. Thank you for your goodness and your blessings. You are a good God. I love you Lord with all my heart, mind, soul, might and strength. You are my God and You loved me. Thank You Jesus, thank You Lord. I will always appreciate what you have done for me and I thank You for Your goodness.*

Thank You for Your tangible presence with me tonight. Thank You for telling me that as I walk with You, and do not lean in my own understanding in everything that I do, I shall receive my complete healing for my mental illness. Thank You Jesus, thank You Lord!

Thank You I am healed in Jesus' name. Lord, I shall walk with you closely and not lean in my own understanding to do what I want to do. Please help me to attain this. Thank You Jesus, thank You Lord! I shall obey You at all times and not grieved the Holy Spirit or missed His voice when He speaks to me. Help me Lord to be sensitive to Your leading, and to always wait upon You to guide and direct my path. I want to be obedient to You and I want to serve You fervently. I will obey You and I will walk with You Intimately and do all that You said to me. Help me to attain doing this in Jesus' name. Thank You Jesus, thank You Lord!

April 15 2013
Awarded at IMH

1st February, 2013 I was warded at IMH. I stayed there the longest in all my stay at IMH since 1984. I was there for more than a month. I was discharged on March 12, 2013 and missed Chinese New Year in February. It was more of a spiritual and physical healing for my mental mind. I was warded at the ICU Ward 80B, where I was alone in a room all by myself. They accused me of not eating, put a tube into my nostril and fed me with milk through the tube. I was also awarded in the ordinary ward, Ward 32, and every day I did nothing, just ate and slept.

After I came back, I felt healed in Jesus' name. My spirit being was exuberant and I was free in my spirit to relate to people. I felt liberated to go and buy Her World magazine, where the Lord told me that I will write for the magazine. I had purposed to go to Kinokuniya at 8 pm, but ended up at NTUC outside my house browsing through the magazines. I could not find Her World but managed to buy it at 7-11.

May 21, 2013
Beginning of my walk with God – Always be with Him

Today I discovered that this is the breakthrough week as I yield to the Lord and be willing to do nothing but to wait on Him. Simply doing nothing and waiting upon Him was what the Lord taught me. In the past, I was frantic that I must be doing something all the time, and out of my own self effort. I am so glad that God has trained me to wait upon Him, as I can be doing nothing and it does not hurt anymore. *Thank You Papa God for making it possible for me to walk with You. I can now commune with You all the time without going my own way or doing my own thing. Every moment with You is beautiful Oh Lord. I enjoy waiting upon You, doing nothing. Thanks for the breakthrough and I am so thankful that You make it possible for me to be transformed*

and be the daughter that You wanted me to be. Thank
You Papa God.

May 9, 2018
Prophetic Conference

The Remember Moses Prophetic Conference on 25
-27 April at Harvester Community Church at Lorong
19, Sims Avenue, was a good time of learning who Moses
was. The three days conference speakers were Prophet
Sadhu Sundar Selvaraj and Pastor Steven Francis. On
the final day of the conference, we had an impartation
by Bro Sadhu in receiving the Moses anointing. I was
slain on my own and God touched me as I found myself
completely liberated and free. The anointing made me
a new person as I felt confident and positive.

On Saturday 5th May, as during the service, I
operated in spiritual gifting as I could discern a man
who needed to get right with God as the altar call was
given to those who needed to repent of their sins. The
Holy Spirit guided me to pray and weep for this soul,
as I felt the compassion of Jesus for this man. Thank
God this man repented and was reconciled with God
again. Hallelujah.

I thank God for my breakthrough, as I now could
hear God clearly, and on 30th April as I went window
shopping, Papa God was present to commune with me
in a very clear voice and strong intimacy with Him. I
enjoyed the conversation with Him and Papa God said

that He enjoyed shopping with me. What a privilege for the Creator God to say this to me. It was really good to hear that. *(I love you Papa God)*. I thank God that He spoke so clearly to me. Glory to God.

25th October 2016
Bee Lan's Demised

I miss my eldest sister Bee Lan, as she had gone home to be with the Lord on 25th October. I will not forget those times when she helped me, like in 2014 when she assisted me to IMH when I was sicked by calling the ambulance and paying $150 for the service. As I was not well, I treated her badly by abusing her with words because in my mind I believe was not sick and she had to take me to the hospital. At the hospital I realised my behaviour, and just before she left home, I apologise to her for my bad behaviour.

Her presence was all it takes to speak of who she was – helpful. She assisted me in the change of my IC, accompanied me to see my doctor every month for the last 4 years since 2012, gave me things, e.g., stockings, (which I still have plenty). She gave me about 2 or more dresses, bought a pyjama for me in 2009, gave me a bottle of perfume, and always did favours for me. I am so glad that she was saved and is now with God and Jesus. I thank God I did not give up on her faith while she was at the hospital, as she said the sinner's prayer with me sometime about 4 months ago before she passed away.

July 26, 2019
My Delayed Healing

I just came back from IMH for my 3-weekly appointment. In the bus I prayed for healing for my arthritis (both knee caps). I earnestly prayed for healing till I came home. I remembered the verses I learnt for healing and quoted them to the Lord. Then the Lord led me to Psalm 103:15-18 where it says that "as for man, his days are like grass; as a flower of the field, so he flourishes. For the wind passes over it, and it is gone, and its place remembers it no more. But the mercy of the Lord is from everlasting to everlasting on those who fear Him, and His righteousness to children's children, to such as keep His covenant, and to those who remember His commandments to do them."

I recalled those time earlier in my calling where God gave me a covenant with Him, which is to minister to people as I have a calling to be an evangelist. I am now 58 (3 days to my 59 birthday), and I am still not serving the Lord yet. The Lord said out of not knowing how to hear Him, I missed my calling. Yes, many times I disobeyed the Lord; even when I turned 40, where God gave me an assignment to minister to the pastors in Singapore. I started the Pastors' Networking in Missions ministry; where the pastors met to serve each other in world missions. I served for about two years from 2004 to 2006 but stepped down because I was in the flesh and did not know how to do the ministry.

The Lord meant for me this year to do ministry, but again I blew it away when I operated in the flesh. I did not pray and commit to the Lord the New Year, and was reprimanded by the Lord for the flesh and could not serve at CornerStone because I was not ready. In the past I did not take time to pray for my healing but I repented and chose to pray daily. I intend to spend my time seeking the Lord, talking to Him about this mountain, be thou be removed and be cast into the sea and does not doubt in my heart but believe that those things I said will come to pass, I'll have whatever I said. (Mk 11:22-23). I claim these verses for myself, that I will not doubt what God said about my healing, and believes that He has already healed me. God is not a God that He should lie, nor a man that He should repent, has He not said it and shall it not come to pass? I believe what God said to me, that I am healed if I obey Him wholeheartedly. Yes, I tend to go my own way and make my own decision, but I repented and no longer walk in sin. I am a new creation in Christ, old things have passed away, behold all things have become new (2 Cor 5:17).

Lord, I thank You for my healing for all my infirmities. I will continue to seek Your face and wait upon You. Thank You for my healing, as I pray in Jesus mighty name. Amen!

10 August 2020
New Lease of Life

Received my healing tonight. Felt a new beginning, able to talk to the Lord exuberantly. Thanking God for my healing after 36 years of mental illness. The Lord is good. He healed me. Thanked You Papa God.

I look forward to my new lease of life. I can begin to have works, read God's Word and have daily routine – writing, reading the Bible, read books, write my novel and start writing blogs.

The Hurdle to the Next Lap

I am so glad with my Papa God who has healed me from schizophrenia. I can now patiently work through the next lap of my hurdle, and that is the goal of seeing the world saved in world evangelisation.

I have a calling to be an evangelist. My desire is that the world will become a better place, as gross darkness is covering the earth now, with the pandemic and other more dangerous traits of variants that will emerge. We see in Isaiah 60:2 that "behold the darkness shall cover the earth, and deep darkness the people." This pandemic is the birth pang of the ends of the world; that Jesus will come back soon into this world for His bride. The world is getting darker and darker, but at the same time, the light of God will shine forth in its majestic glory as Jesus is coming back. The return of Jesus in

His second coming will be a glorious event, as the whole world will witness His coming onto the clouds of glory.

Since I am healed from my mental illness, my next hurdle will be world evangelisation. The world is in need of direction and purpose, those who cannot see the hind sight of their future will face a gigantic hurdle of bread-and-butter issue, far beyond than what they can imagine. The security of the once prosperous status will crumble, and you will not be able to see the other side of the rainbow in your own turf. Pressing issues of your present situation cannot be compared with the more heinous circumstances that you will find yourself in.

So, what is becoming of the world does involve you and me. The only security that one can look to is none other than the creator of this world who made heaven and earth. God created this world for His pleasure. What the enemy has stolen, Jesus has already claimed it back on Calvary cross 2,000 years ago. Jesus first coming was to redeem the world back to Himself. He suffered a cruel death so that He can redeem mankind back to Himself. The crucifixion of Jesus was the most glandulous of human history, as He conquered the world through His blood that was shed for you and me, to receive the penalty and the guilt of mankind upon Himself. Jesus' mission was simply to bring mankind back to God, where our Creator God created this world and it will return back to Him when Jesus comes back again. This world is temporary, our greater inheritance is not in this world but in the next world to come. God is seated at His throne and He will claim the world back to Himself.

If you are facing anguish and pain right now, know that Jesus our redeemer has already claimed the victory for you. All you have to do is just to accept Jesus into your life. He is the maker of this world, and He knows exactly what you need. Will you accept Jesus into your life right now; will you call upon Him to save you from all your setbacks and pains? Call upon Him now and you shall be saved. Jesus is calling you back home. Your real home is in heaven; He has prepared a place for you if you were to accept Him as your personal Lord and saviour. Salvation is free in Jesus because He has already paid the price for your sins on the cross. All you have to do is to believe in Jesus and accept Him into your life. Cry out to Him now and He will take you into His arm just as you are. Wait no more for this free gift in Jesus.

If you would like to accept Jesus into your life or you have already acknowledged Him as you saviour, then pray this prayer aloud to yourself:

Jesus, I thank You that You are the source of Life. Thank you for dying on the cross for my sin. I know You are God and I want to accept You into my life. Come into my heart as I accept You as my personal Lord and saviour. Thank You for redeeming me for the blood that you shed on the cross. I welcome You into my life and take me as I am. In Jesus most precious and holy name I pray, Amen!

Glory hallelujah! If you have prayed this prayer, know that your sins are washed and forgiven. You are now a child of God. Welcome to the family of God.

If you would like to know more about Jesus and how you can grow in this faith, or you have questions that you like answered, please email me. My email is: delinetan29@gmail.com